A CUP OF COMFORT®
for Families Touched by
Alzheimer's

Inspirational stories of
unconditional love
and support

Edited by Colleen Sell

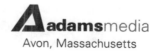
Adamsmedia
Avon, Massachusetts

In loving memory of Mary Louise Baum

A *Cup of Comfort*® is a registered trademark of F+W Publications, Inc.

Published by
Adams Media, an F+W Publications Company
57 Littlefield Street, Avon, MA 02322 U.S.A.
www.adamsmedia.com and *www.cupofcomfort.com*

ISBN-10: 1-59869-651-3
ISBN-13: 978-1-59869-651-6
Printed in the United States of America.

J I H G F E D C B A

Library of Congress Cataloging-in-Publication Data
is available from the publisher.

This publication is designed to provide accurate and authoritative information with regard to the subject matter covered. It is sold with the
understanding that the publisher is not engaged in rendering legal,
accounting, or other professional advice. If legal advice or other expert
assistance is required, the services of a competent professional person
should be sought.

—From a *Declaration of Principles* jointly adopted by
a Committee of the American Bar Association and
a Committee of Publishers and Associations

Many of the designations used by manufacturers and sellers to distin-
guish their products are claimed as trademarks. Where those designations appear in this book and Adams Media was aware of a trademark
claim, the designations have been printed with initial capital letters.

This book is available at quantity discounts for bulk purchases.
For information, please call 1-800-289-0963.

Contents

Acknowledgments

First, I wish to express my love and gratitude for my maternal grandmother, Mary Louise Baum, whose presence in my life helped me to better understand dementia and to feel compassion, respect, and affection for those held in its grip. I miss her fiercely—quirks and all.

I am most grateful to the authors whose stories grace the pages of this book, for sharing these extraordinary chapters of their lives. A nod of appreciation also goes to the more than 2,000 people whose stories did not make it into this book. It is not easy to write about the very personal and sometimes painful experiences of living with and losing a loved one with Alzheimer's—much less to do so in a way that brings comfort to others. Bravo. And bless you all.

A boatload of thanks goes to the outstanding crew at Adams Media—especially to Meredith O'Hayre (expert navigator), Laura Daly (stalwart skipper), Paula Munier (visionary captain), and deckhands extraordinaire, Carol Goff and Jacquinn Williams.

Introduction

"If my hands are fully occupied in holding on to something, I can neither give nor receive."

—*Dorothee Sölle*

An estimated 26 million people worldwide and more than 4.5 million Americans have Alzheimer's disease (AD)—a progressive, degenerative brain disorder that leads to dementia and death. Although genetics and cognitive deficits earlier in life may play a role in Alzheimer's, it is the development of lesions on the brain, called "senile plaques" and "neurofibrillary tangles," that signal the onset and determine the severity of Alzheimer's. Symptoms usually become noticeable between the ages of sixty-five and eighty-five but can arise as early as age forty-five, and the disease can take from two to twenty years to run its course. Alzheimer's has no known cause or cure, and so, at least for now, treatment consists of minimizing the symptoms and providing support to people with Alzheimer's and their families, who are often caregivers for at least a portion of their loved ones' journey with the disease.

As prevalent as Alzheimer's is—and the number is expected to grow to 106 million people by 2050—it is still a shock when it is your beloved parent, partner, grandparent, or sibling whose mind begins to fail or who is diagnosed with AD. As good as the medical and care providers; social services; and support of family, friends, and community might be, it is never enough to offset the emotional, physical, and financial toll on people with AD and their families. As promising as the scientific research is that one day we will have effective treatment and perhaps even a cure for Alzheimer's, today it is still a terminal disease.

So it is understandable that most of us think of Alzheimer's with dread and despair. It is no wonder that, when a loved one is diagnosed with AD, we often cling to what was and fear what will be. And it is only human to become so overwhelmed with the heartbreaking realities and crushing responsibilities of this disease that we miss opportunities to comfort and to connect with our loved one with Alzheimer's. Sometimes we even overlook the joys and blessings they bring.

The extraordinary essays gathered here in *A Cup of Comfort for Families Touched by Alzheimer's* provide an intimate window inside the lives and hearts of those who have gone before us and who are now walking with us on the journey through Alzheimer's disease. These inspiring stories focus not on the trials and tragedies of AD (though, neither do they whitewash those realities), but rather on the gifts that individuals have given and received during their personal journeys with Alzheimer's. I hope, and trust, that these stories will bring you great comfort and will inspire you to give comfort to your fellow travelers on this incredible journey.

—*Colleen Sell*

Only Love Remains

Who was this little old man hobbling along beside me? He may have been wondering the same thing: Who is this woman walking beside me? Yet, he seemed to know one thing for sure: I was going to take him to see his sweetheart, his bride of sixty-four years. So he was working as hard as he could to put one foot in front of the other as we exited the Alzheimer's center. He willingly—no, eagerly—eased himself into the passenger seat of my car, looking up at me hopefully through clouded, blue eyes.

After I'd helped Dad buckle his seat belt, I wasn't sure what to say as we drove toward the hospital. I wasn't certain if his old ears could even hear me. And if he did hear, I wasn't sure how much he could comprehend. I decided to talk about Mom. I knew she was his only goal, the only person he could remember. The staff at the center told me Dad hadn't slept all night. Instead, he'd sat near the reception desk, hoping the front door would open and the love of his life would return to him. He couldn't function without Mom around.

"She's doing okay, Dad," I shouted, so I might be heard.

The old man's face brightened, so I continued.

"The hospital told me they're releasing her today because she has only a minor problem, gout, I think. They just wanted to keep her overnight for observation. But she sure scared us last night with those tremors, didn't she?"

Dad just looked confused and stared at me fearfully. After a while he turned away, looking puzzled. I guess I shouldn't have said that. He obviously didn't remember last night—Mom's nearly convulsive tremors and our ride to the hospital. I shouldn't have mentioned it. I didn't want to upset him. He didn't need any more stress right now. It was stress enough to have spent the night without his bride.

I never knew what to say to Dad. He said very little. When he did try to speak, his words came out slowly, a jumble of random thoughts. And he had to work really hard when he spoke. He worked so hard at putting words together and would be so satisfied at having said something. I'd learned to just nod and smile, as if

I knew what point he was trying to make. Most of the time, I had no clue and I wondered if he did.

I wanted to cry. I fought the urge by taking a journey back in time to a day thirty-five years earlier, when I'd volunteered to help Dad pick out a Christmas gift for Mom. As we walked the city streets at his athletic pace, one person after another would call out, "Hi, Judge!" Some greeted him warmly, as friends. Others kowtowed as if he were royalty. Regardless, Dad reached out to everyone with broad smiles, warm handshakes, and questions about their families. He seemed to know the entire population of this little city! I was proud to be walking beside this man, my new father-in-law, the "Judge."

He'd been on the bench as a superior court judge for more than twenty years at that point. Very few folks regarded Dad as an enemy because he had a way of winning their hearts with his outgoing nature and generosity. I nearly burst with pride when a man of about forty marched up and thanked Dad for throwing him in prison years earlier. "Judge," he declared, smiling from ear to ear, "you really did me a favor. Getting locked up in jail was the best thing that ever happened to me. It gave me a new start. You knew just what I needed."

The "Judge" was the man I remembered, not this shriveled old man beside me who looked weak and vulnerable. Although his wife still insisted he be addressed as "Judge," this wasn't the same man. An occasional grin would light his face and remind me of him, but the Judge was gone.

His bride was in a similar condition. She still went about like the proverbial schoolteacher, correcting everyone's English and etiquette. And she played bridge marvelously, according to her old bridge club. Yet, her mind had failed to retain much else after her last surviving child, my husband, passed away three years earlier at age fifty-six from complications of multiple sclerosis.

"John?" she often calls, "John?"—as if she could summon him back to her side.

It had been difficult enough when John's older brother had drowned at the age of thirty. We hadn't been sure Mom would survive it. But when Mom lost John, she also lost her grasp on reality. So she and Dad lived in a room together at the Alzheimer's center. Day after day, they sat dozing side by side in their recliners in front of their television, only leaving the room for meals. It was very much the same as they'd been doing at home, except that they'd become a danger to themselves living alone. Now their lives were reduced to bare-bones survival and total dependence.

I drove the rest of the way to the hospital in silence. I couldn't think of a thing to say that would

comfort my father-in-law more than actually seeing his bride. I'd had to lock the car doors as we
drove along, because Dad had begun to fuss with
the handle. Maybe he hoped Mom was just beyond
the open door. Once I'd found a parking spot at
the hospital and released the lock, Dad immediately
tried to escape. I unfastened his seat belt and eased it
over him. Then we were off, at a snail's pace for me,
but Dad was plodding faster than I'd seen him go in
months.

Once we'd entered the elevator, he fidgeted nervously with the buttons on his sweater. He hardly
knew what to do with himself. When we arrived on
Mom's floor, Dad nearly leaped to be beside me as we
exited the elevator. His eyes were trained on me, so
he wouldn't miss a turn as we wound our way around
corners to Mom's room.

"This is it," I said pointing. "Mom's in there."

Dad virtually ran to her bed! The instant she saw
him, she reached up with one arm to welcome him.
Joy shone from her wrinkled face. Before I knew it,
Dad had settled his cheek into Mom's upraised hand
and was gazing contentedly into her eyes. For one
long moment, those two were frozen in that pos-
ture, unblinking, as they looked with longing at one
another. It was as if I could see decades of memories
flying between them.

Suddenly embarrassed, as if I were trespassing on a most intimate scene, I turned and walked to the window. As I stared blankly into space, I was trying to process what I'd just seen. I knew my in-laws had become closer as they'd grown older, but this didn't seem like the same couple I'd known for thirty-eight years. They used to fight like cats and dogs, used to pick at each other's faults, used to squabble over the rule of the home and remote control. So what was this? John and I had always hoped these two would declare a truce and realize the treasure they had in one another. What had happened? I wasn't sure, at first, but whatever it was, it was wonderful.

Then I began to think back to the day when my husband had been diagnosed with multiple sclerosis. Suddenly, he became the most precious thing in this world. The very thought of losing John was unbearable. Our love only grew stronger during the thirty years of John's increasing disability. We focused intensely on the blessings we had each moment of each day, because we never knew when we would have to say good-bye. The last words we'd exchanged were "I love you."

Now, it was my in-laws' turn. Their bodies were failing, their minds were nearly gone, and their children had preceded them in death. Yet, at the end of it all, they'd discovered riches beyond comprehension. They'd discovered the value in one another.

Still gazing out the hospital window, I smiled to myself as I heard Mom speaking softly to Dad with sweet, soothing words. I doubted he could hear her, but I knew he was watching intently as her lips moved. He loved those lips. He loved that woman as he loved himself—perhaps even more. That's all he knew. That's all he needed to know. Everything else in his life was gone, only love remained.

—Laura L. Bradford

Lost in the Moment

"I'm going to kill you!" he yells, drawing his arm back and forming a fist.

I hurry to unlock the car, and suddenly he is yanking on my brown ponytail, jerking my head backward. "Stop! You're hurting me!" I yell as he pulls harder. Reaching behind me, I try to grab him and peel myself away from this skinny, gray-haired man. Instead, he takes my arm and twists it back toward him. I wince as I feel his teeth sink hard into the back of my hand. Using a force reserved for times when I am really feeling physically threatened, I sink my fingernails deep into his bony shoulder. Stunned, he drops his arms to his sides and looks at me like he doesn't know what to do next. A black SUV slows to a stop a few feet away.

"Are you okay?" a woman who looks to be about fifty calls to me.

"Yes," I tell her, huffing, wishing she would just leave.

"Are you sure?" she asks, sounding unconvinced.

"Everything is fine," I say, feeling heat rise to my face. It is bad enough when this happens at home. "It's Alzheimer's."

"Oh," she says and pauses, then drives away, leaving us standing there, spilled groceries strewn around our feet on the wet pavement.

I hold my father firmly by the shoulders and look straight into his gray-blue eyes. "It's me, Laurie. I'm your daughter," I say. "This really is our car. You're safe."

He stares at me blankly, and then I feel his body soften as he seems to experience some flash of recognition. I help him get seated on the waterproof pad and fasten his seatbelt. "Thank you very much," he says with a grateful smile, as though nothing has happened.

Waiting at a red light, rain patters on the windshield, and the heater has just started blowing warm air on our feet. My father has fallen fast asleep and is snoring softly. His tousled hair looks especially white against his royal blue parka. His head is bent toward his left shoulder, and his large knuckled fingers lay limp on his lap. A tiny pool of drool is forming on the seatbelt that crosses his sunken chest.

My hand throbs. I trace a finger around the ring of purple teeth marks and wonder how we got to this place, my father and I. Where have the ten years gone since my mother died? When did this disease intercept his grief over her death so that he no longer remembers that she was ever here at all? When did I become the parent and he the child?

At five feet eleven inches and 135 pounds and with eighty-five years of life behind him, my father is so frail it would seem that just a whisper of wind could knock him over, if not do him in completely. Yet, when he strikes out, it seems to be fueled by a fear so primal that no reason can quell it. When the world seems to be spinning out of control for me, I have to remind myself that for him it is spinning far faster. He is merely struggling to survive it.

I hit the preprogrammed button on my car radio—"home of the oldies" comes on, and I turn up the volume. It's James Taylor, the Beatles, and the Stones. When did the music from my youth become that of the distant past? Did I really spend years at a university, complete a master's degree, travel the world, and have a career? I see the slight bounce of my father's knee out of the corner of my eye. Mick Jagger's singing, which years ago he would have shunned, now brings him to life.

My father starts clapping and humming, hitting the dash in rhythm to the beat of "Get Off My Cloud." Dad waves and smiles at people in passing cars, as if they should be able to hear the uplifting music too. I am laughing, caught up in his joy, when he grabs my hand from the steering wheel and pulls it toward his mouth. My stomach flips as I try to keep my eyes on the road. The sting still lingers from earlier, and I ready myself for what he might do next. Then he draws my hand to his lips and softly kisses the back of it. For a second, our eyes meet, and I have the father I remember back with me.

"I love you!" he declares. "I love you, Laur-ie!" he repeats, sweeping upward with the last syllable of my name as he turns away and looks out the window.

Anxious to ride this wave of carefree energy, I pull into a McDonald's drive-through and order a large strawberry shake. This sudden lightheartedness might make him feel like downing some serious calories. I scold myself for not searching out something more nutritious, but by the time I find it, this good mood could well have passed. *Just get some food into him,* I tell myself, *anything to counteract the alarming effects of his dwindling appetite.*

"Would you like some ice cream?" I ask as we wait in line.

"That sounds good!" he says with an innocence that makes me want to protect him.

"Look here!" he says, pointing to his window as it lowers. He pushes the button on his armrest again, and the window goes back up.

"Did you see that?" he asks, looking utterly perplexed.

He pushes it again, and the window lowers again to the sound of his laughter.

I drive forward, the blue-uniformed girl hands me the milkshake, and I pass it over to him. As I turn to ask her for a napkin, my father suddenly yells, "I don't want this. Why did you give me this?"

"It's your favorite. Just taste it," I coax.

"I don't want it!" he yells.

Resigned, I reach for the cup, but he won't let me have it. Drawing his arm back, his fingers squeeze the paper cup so hard it is starting to spill over the top. When riled, my father will sometimes pick up whatever is close at hand and throw it at me, and he will throw with all his might.

"Please, let me take it," I force my tone to sound as soothing as possible, knowing it is my only hope for diffusing this moment.

"No! You can't have it!" he shouts back, venom in his voice, and takes aim. I grab for the cup, and he clenches it harder. Now we are engaged in a precarious game of tug-of-war with the slippery cup. My father wins and hurls the cup at me. The flimsy plastic lid flies off, and the milkshake explodes all over me. The pink liquid drips all through my hair, down my face and shirt, onto my lap and quickly forms sticky streams between the ridges on the rubber mat beneath my feet. The cloyingly sweet smell and the sadness of the situation turn my stomach.

"Why did you do that?" I ask, unable to hide my despair.

"I don't want it!" he repeats, his eyes wide with ire.

The girl at the window stares at us, expressionless. "Alzheimer's," I say, as she hands me a wad of napkins and turns away.

I pull into the disabled parking space and pop the trunk. Pushing aside the extra Depends and pants that I carry everywhere "just in case," I search around the damp grocery bags for my gym clothes. In the restroom, I lock the door and sink to the cold, brick-color tiled floor. Tears rise from a place normally forced into submission, and I fight the urge to let them keep coming. But now is not the time.

"Breathe," I say out loud to myself. I force myself to pull in some air and stand up. Leaning against the wall for support, I feel lightheaded and lost. Rinsing the sticky mess out of my hair and splashing my face, I watch the water turn pink as it swirls around the drain with my tears and disappears. I change my clothes and hurry back outside and feel relief when I see the white-haired figure napping in the front seat. At least it will not be one of those days when I let down my guard and he wanders away. It will not be one of those panicked times when the police and I search together frantically for this lost man. Yes, it could have been worse.

"Let's go!" my father says, all smiles, when I resume my position in the driver's seat. "Go that way!" he directs, pointing with the authoritative tone of someone who once ran a large company.

I turn to the right. What difference does it make to me? If it gives him a feeling of being in control while the disease continues to relentlessly steal what little he has left, then why not. My goal today, like every day, is simply to get him out of the house so that he can see the world and still feel a part of it. Even if he doesn't know that this is the city in which he has lived for sixty years. Even if he uses words I don't always understand. Even if he doesn't know that I am his daughter.

Following my father's whims, we weave our way across town. We are stopped at a red light with cars driving fast across our bow when he yells, "Go!"

"I have to wait for the light to turn green," I say.

"No, you don't. Go!" he shouts again.

I lean my head back against the headrest, muster the energy to draw in another deep breath, and wait out the light and his protestations.

Today he seems a little more unpredictable than usual, quicker to agitate. I could give him the pills that I keep in my purse for such situations, but I hate to use them because they make him so sleepy that we don't get to connect at all. I would rather put up with the difficult moments so that I don't have to miss the sweet ones, for those are the ones that keep me going. It is a choice that I consciously make even though I have the occasional bruise and the occasional meltdown of my own. I watch the window of our time together closing moment by moment, and I never know when a flash of lucidity will hit. I want to be ready to embrace it when it does, for it is all I have left of the father I once knew and the relationship we once had.

Continuing on, we head out on a bridge that crosses a large lake behind the city. His head turns left, right, and up to the sky, and I watch him trace a plane as it fades into the clouds.

"Look at that!" he says excitedly.

I glance around and see water, mountains, boats—the usual.

"What do you see that's so special?" I ask.

"Look! All of it!" he exclaims, stretching his arms outward like a guide, showing me the magic of creation. He leans forward to get closer to the windshield to gain a better view. His eyes are bright, and his laughter fills the space we share.

It is as if my father is five, not eighty-five, and is seeing the world for the first time. I think of my countless yoga and meditation classes, of all the self-help books I have read over the years, of all my attempts to "live mindfully" and to "be here now." Yet, here is my father, bearing the burden of an insidious and devastating disease, fully alive in the moment. Unable to recall the past or to conceive of the future, he does not waste time on regret or worry.

"It's beautiful! It's absolutely beautiful! Don't you see it?"

While much of the meaning of the catch phrase "living in the moment" has been lost to triteness, for the Alzheimer's victim it is a way of life. My father resides in the present because it is all that he has left. While I cling to memories of how things used to be and reach out longingly with hope for the future, my father shows me every day that it is in the place between these two that life is really happening. Ironically, it is we who have the ability to remember who too easily forget this basic truth.

—*Laurie McConnachie*

Wanted: Another Mother

"Okay, Mom, I've had enough," I say, standing up and crossing my arms across my chest. "Really, if you don't start paying more attention to me, I'm going to have to do something drastic. I'm going to have to find another mother. Mom, are you listening? Mom?"

Mom is definitely not listening, which is, of course, part of the problem.

I walk out of the Alzheimer's unit, my hands clenched and my jaw tight. Of course, I knew this would happen. I understand the progression of the disease. What I didn't understand is how much I would miss having a mother.

I get into the car, feeling like a small child having a big fit. I realize that if I want any semblance of the sort of mother figure I am used to, I will have to go out and find her. I am not going to abandon my own mother; I just want to supplement her.

I envision my personal ad:

MAD desires OM for LTR. (Middle-Aged Daughter desires Other Mother for Long-Term Relationship.) Seeking bright, opinionated, literate, compassionate, older woman. Must be a good listener. A propensity for sweets preferred.

I know there are wonderful adoption programs for older children who need good homes. Is there a venue for midlife women who are either orphaned or feel motherless? Perhaps some entrepreneurial Internet expert can put together match-dot-mom. Perhaps instead of the adopt-a-grandparent program in the schools, the retirement centers and nursing homes can advocate an adopt-a-daughter program. Wouldn't some lonely elder goddess-crone enjoy having me as her surrogate child?

At the grocery store, I study the women as I push my cart down the aisles. What kind of mother do I want? Do I want a mother in the proper age range, or will a loving, motherly woman my own age or slightly older do? Is body type an issue? My own mother is slender, but perhaps this time I want a plus-size mom. And what of personality? My mother is a great listener, always eager to hear another person's issues and thoughts. Is that a requirement? Mom also has a lot of rules and opinions. Is a woman who likes to be in control a necessity?

For the next few weeks, as I go to meetings and gatherings and run errands, I find myself gazing at older women and wondering, *Would you like to be my other mother?*

Right away, I find several excellent candidates. One friend's mom, in her eighties, is an avid volunteer, card player, and reader. She is kind and thoughtful and also opinionated in a way similar to my mom. Another friend, who spent her seventy-fifth birthday camping in the Saharan desert, would make an adventuresome and outgoing mother. Yet another friend, only in her mid-sixties, has warmth and compassion as well as a gift for baking; I imagine what a cozy, comforting mom she would make.

I decide to treat the other-mother-selection process like I am filling a high-powered job. I create an interview form featuring questions such as:

What makes a good mother-daughter relationship?

How many daughters do you currently have? (I didn't want too much competition.)

What is your definition of success?

What do you like to read?

What kinds of topics do you like to talk about?

What special qualities do you have to offer as my other-mother?

I imagine inviting each potential mother figure to lunch, my questions at the ready. I imagine they all have excellent listening skills, compassion, wit, and appropriate interest in arts and literature. They each answer easily, forthrightly, with focus and thoughtfulness. They are nicely dressed, health conscious without being fanatical, and easy to be around. I would have no problem claiming any one of them as one of my most important relatives.

"How's it coming with the search for your new mother?" a friend asks. Her own mother died some years ago, and she is watching me closely, in case my idea turns out to be a good one.

"I have three amazing candidates, but something's missing. I can't figure out what," I tell her.

Meanwhile, I visit my real mom. I note the contrast: instead of meeting a well-groomed articulate woman at a nice restaurant, I punch a red button and enter the locked Alzheimer's ward.

Louise, a new patient, walks toward me.

"Hello," I say as she rushes up.

"Oh, hello. I'm so happy to see you. I don't know what I'm supposed to be doing," she says. Her cheeks are the flush of new roses. Her pink sweater is clean and properly buttoned.

Is this my other mother? I wonder briefly.

She walks to the dining room with me. Then I look around for Mom.

My mom is in her room, asleep, angled across the bed with her feet on the ground. I watch her for a while, and then I tap her leg. She opens her eyes. I wave at her. She smiles. I wave harder.

She laughs. The anxiety that sometimes grips her, causing her to rub her hands against her head or to yank at her clothes, has temporarily melted away. She is simply a beautiful, silver-haired woman on a summer day.

I keep silent and look into my mom's eyes. She looks into my eyes. The air is pure and sweet between us. There is no misunderstanding, no lost thoughts, no forced or garbled sentences. We are two creatures gazing at each other with openness and compassion. I hear the nurse aides going about their work, the patients walking down the corridor. I hear the large cart that carries the lunch dishes rumble down the hallway. But those sounds are background music—I am connected only with my mother.

As I look into her eyes, I wonder, *What makes us walk away from our mothers and then run back? What makes us pretend we are not our mothers—that we have nothing in common with these women? What lets us imagine we are going to be so much stronger, smarter, and happier than they were?*

I have spent a lot of time separating myself from my mother. Now, I want to be closer.

I sink into my mother's face like she is a meditation. We smile at each other for a half hour, something we have never done before, something that would be too intense, too personal, in our earlier, rational life together.

Then her eyes gently flutter shut. I feel like I've been on a mystical retreat. I feel a rich sense of renewal and hope.

As I watch my mother fall into slumber, I realize I don't really want another mother. I like the softer, less-controlled persona of this mother. I like her silly noises and ready laughter. I like the fact that she doesn't know who I am but smiles at me anyway. I am growing comfortable with her new, unorthodox style of motherhood.

Mom's eyes are closed; her hands rest by her sides. I kneel on the floor and rest my head against her legs. I feel her warmth and the sureness of her breathing. Then I feel her hand on my head, tugging playfully at my curls, just like she used to do when I was a little girl. I smile, close my eyes, and rest.

—*Deborah Shouse*

This story was first published in the author's book, Love in the Land of Dementia: Finding Hope in the Caregiver's Journey, *Creativity Connection Press, August 2006.*

You're Going the Wrong Way

Jim taps me on the face. "Honey, honey, you're going the wrong way," he says.

I open my eyes and glance at the clock. It is 4:00 A.M. Jim stands beside me, wearing his jacket, his shoes, and underwear. "You need to put on your jeans," I tell him, squeezing my eyelids shut.

"Honey, you're going the wrong way," he tells me.

"Let me sleep just a little longer," I say. I may be whining a bit out of exhaustion, because he wouldn't go to sleep before midnight last night. My arms and legs feel heavy; my eyes are tired and gritty. Working full-time and being a primary caregiver for my husband shrouds my life with a fog of exhaustion. Stress is a small word to describe the physical demands of caregiving and the emotional drain of coping with the declining cognizance of my soul mate.

I hear the buzz of the electric razor as Jim shaves. "You're going the wrong way!" Jim is back, and he sounds cranky.

I open one eye. Now, he is dressed in his jacket, shoes, and socks, sans underwear, unconcerned with his nakedness. I toss the covers aside and jump out of bed to help him, because, obviously, today he is unable to dress himself.

I yank loose the Velcro on his shoes. After Jim removes his shoes, I hand him cotton boxers, and he slowly puts them on. He pulls on 501 Levis, and I button them, which is not an easy task. I hand him his shoes, and he slides his feet into them. He is already wearing his denim jacket, complete with a Branson Veteran's Day nametag and scatter pins.

Once Jim is fully dressed, it's time to make coffee and start the day. Now, it's five o'clock, so it doesn't seem so much like we're getting up in the middle of the night. In the kitchen, I discover Jim has already started the coffee. Coffee has run all over the counter and onto the kitchen carpet, because he neglected to place the carafe beneath the basket. I clean up the mess and brew a second pot.

After breakfast, it's time for Jim's meds. I pour the correct dosage out of the bottles and place the pills in his hand. I open the refrigerator and reach for his water. Jim pops the pills into his mouth, and before

I can give him a drink, he spits them back out. Jim licks the soggy pills from his hand and takes a tiny sip of water to wash them down.

I feed our two big dogs and hand Jim a can of dog food for the beagle. He opens the door and heads outside carrying the can.

"Wait!" I say. "You have to open the can."

Jim wanders back into the kitchen, clutching the can and looking around with a blank expression on his face.

I open a drawer and hand him a can opener. "Here, use this."

He opens the can, and as he goes out the door, I walk into the bedroom to get dressed. I return to the kitchen to find dog food dumped into the sink. I scrape it up, spoon it back into the can, and feed the hungry-eyed beagle standing at the door.

Jim opens the doors to the entertainment center and drags his Super Nintendo out onto the floor. He sits on his knees like a child and throws me a challenging look.

"I don't want to play," I say. I know the game will be Mario Karts. That's the only game I can even come close to playing. I'm no good at it, and Jim always wins.

He ignores my protests and pushes the start button. I pick up a control as he zips through the game selections. As usual, he is Toad.

"Who should my driver be?"

"Princess," he says. I smile, because this is always his suggestion. He used to call me Princess.

The track is before us, and we sit on the start line. The game begins, and Toad zooms away while I fumble with the control, trying to figure out how to get Princess on the road. Finally, I get Princess started, and with my help she runs off the track and spins around corners, and soon a little guy perched on a cloud waves a flag with a big "X" on it.

"You're going the wrong way!" Jim shouts with glee.

"I know, I know!" I say, thinking it's not nearly as funny as he thinks it is.

Toad crosses the finish line, and Jim clicks off the game, satisfied that he beat me again.

After the game, he rambles restlessly through the house. As I dust, the front door chimes repeatedly as Jim opens it. I tell him to "come back" if he is outside or to "stay here" if he hasn't actually gone out yet.

Downstairs, I remove laundry from the dryer and fold clothes. The phone rings, and my sister-in-law says, "Jim is on the road in front of our house." Darn! I didn't know he was gone. Sometimes he doesn't close the door completely, and the chimes don't ring. I jump in the car and drive down the gravel road to retrieve him.

After I finish the housework, I decide to take him for a ride. "Let's go to town," I say. I walk to the bedroom to get my purse. The door chimes ding, but I ignore them because I know he will wait by the car. Outside, I don't see Jim, and I think he has wandered off again. I am relieved to find him sitting on the passenger side with his seat belt fastened.

It is a hot summer day, and the windows are rolled up tight. Jim wears his denim jacket, and sweat pours off him. I start the car and turn on the air conditioner full blast, and we are off to town.

Going to town is always an adventure. Jim is all smiles, because traveling makes him happy. The sun shines through the windows and flecks of lint float through the air and collect on the cloth seats, where Jim picks at the tiny pieces. He captures some lint between this thumb and forefinger and reaches over to roll down the window, but instead he grabs the door handle. I brake, pull off the highway, and park on the shoulder. I reach across Jim and close his door. Jim doesn't realize he's done anything wrong.

We go to Ryan's for lunch. I order from the menu, because buffets are entirely too confusing for Jim. The waiter brings our food, and Jim looks at his plate without attempting to eat anything. I put sweetener in his tea and stir it. While I attend to cutting his steak, he drinks the entire glass of tea and wants more. I get the waiter's attention, and he refills the glass. Jim drinks that glass of tea, too, but still hasn't tasted his food. Once the tea glass is empty again, Jim picks up a spoon and attempts to eat the steak with it. I casually snare the spoon and replace it with a fork. I notice other people staring at us, but it doesn't bother me and it certainly doesn't bother Jim. People do not expect a person in his early fifties to have dementia, and many just think he is odd.

We finish our meals and drive across the street to Wal-Mart, Jim's favorite store. Jim makes a beeline to the bathroom. I follow him to the back of the store to make sure he goes into the men's room. I wait and wait and wait. He finally emerges, Levis unbuttoned and belt unbuckled. I button his jeans and fasten his belt, and then we do our shopping.

When we get home twenty minutes later, I park the car, open the trunk, and unload the sacks from Wal-Mart. I can't convince Jim to help carry the bags. Sometimes he will, but today isn't one of those times. Jim wanders to the front door and waits for me to unlock it. I grab the handles of a half dozen plastic sacks, carry them to the porch, and after a struggle with the key, unlock the door. Jim walks into the house, and I toss the first load inside. While I trek back to the garage for the rest of the sacks, Jim carries the first batch into the bedroom. After I figure out where he has put them, I lug them back to the kitchen.

Jim is in the bathroom shaving.

"Hey, we need to walk the dogs," I tell him.

Jim unplugs his razor and tosses it aside. I rush to keep up with him as he jogs down the stairs and opens the patio door.

My German shepherd, Sherry, and Jim's ninety-pound dog, Bubba, bark when we take the leashes off the gate. Their eyes flash with anticipation, and they both indulge in full-body squirming. I fasten Sherry's leash to her collar. Jim has a puzzled look on his face as he holds Bubba's leash, as if he can't figure out what to do with it. While I am distracted with Sherry, Jim opens the gate and walks out carrying Bubba's leash. I grab the hook and fasten it to Bubba's collar.

We take an extra long walk to burn off some of Jim's excess energy. Upon our return, we enter the house through the basement, and I stop to fold laundry before going upstairs. I hear the door chimes, and by the time I climb the stairs, Jim is headed toward the road. I yell at him, and he comes back.

Jim goes to the bathroom and shaves.

I put *Lonesome Dove* in the VCR for Jim to watch. He settles in front of the TV and takes a short nap.

When Jim awakens from his nap, it is early evening and bath time. I run the water and coach Jim in taking off his clothes. I throw all the dirty clothes in the hamper and lead him to the tub.

"Get in the tub," I tell him, and he obediently climbs in.

I shampoo his hair with baby shampoo, soap him up, and rinse him off. He enjoys soaking in the tub, so I decide to brush my teeth. Before I realize it, he is up and out and walking across the bathroom floor, dripping wet. I lead him back to the bath mat and grab a towel off the rack. He stands like a statue while I dry him.

"Here, put these on." I hand him his undershorts, and he slowly puts his feet through the leg holes and pulls up the boxers. I place his T-shirt in his hands, and after he puts it on, he sits on the bathroom floor and slowly pulls on his socks and sweatpants. Finally! He is ready for bed.

Jim settles in front of the TV to watch a *Walker* rerun, and I take my bath. When I emerge from the bathroom, Jim is fully clothed with his jeans over his sweatpants. If I undress him now, he will just dress again, so the best plan is to wait until bedtime.

Jim shaves and forgets to turn off the razor.

At ten o'clock, I give Jim his new nighttime medication, lead him to bed, and remove his clothes.

Jim will soon be sound asleep; then I will have some peace and quiet for about four hours. Tomorrow will bring different challenges as my husband continues to lose the ability to cope with the minutiae of life.

I kiss him on the forehead and tuck the covers around him. I brush my hand across his smooth cheek and breathe in memories along with the scent of his Old Spice cologne. I whisper in his ear, "I love you. But you're going the wrong way."

"Princess," he mumbles, and I wonder if he is thinking of Mario Karts or me. He smiles and drifts off to sleep.

—L. S. Fisher

The Bird House

Grandma Rose has Alzheimer's disease. Her son, Ross, my father, also has Alzheimer's disease. He was diagnosed at age fifty-eight and she at seventy-nine. At the beginning, Grandma understood that her son was very sick, and when she told me her doctor had said that "it was about the worse thing you could get," the last word sounded like a sob. Nearly six months have passed since my father's diagnosis, and in those months, names, dates, facts, and figures have slipped from my grandmother's mind like minnows into a stream.

Grandma Rose has begun to hit people. She's a tiny woman, standing barely five feet tall and weighing just six pounds more than she did on her wedding day. She's always been pretty meek. Hitting is completely out of character. She has also begun to swear. "Shit," she says. Then she goes back to being quiet, staring out at the world through the gold frames of her glasses.

"These frames cost me almost two hundred dollars," she told me once. "They're real nice, aren't they?" Six months ago, she was careful to clean her glasses and careful to stow them in a soft leather case when she wasn't wearing them. Now, the glasses are bent and smudged. The hitting and the swearing are just two more signs that her carefulness is beginning to disappear.

Grandma is living in a nursing home called La Paloma Blanca. The name means "the white dove" and is supposed to conjure up images of peace and calm. My dad always calls it "the bird house," which brings to mind the constant rustle of feathers, the scrape of beak and claw, and seems much more appropriate. The place is big and white with a series of long, linoleum-covered hallways radiating out from a central nurses' hub.

Grandma shares her room with a chatty woman named Doris, who is confined to a wheelchair and delights in windy descriptions of her grandchildren. Grandma's closet is filled with the bright blues and pinks and reds of her exclusively polyester wardrobe. She has a television, a reading lamp, and a framed drawing of her namesake flower, the rose. We hung her crucifix on the wall and pinned photos of distant relations on her bulletin board.

When we visit Grandma Rose, we read letters from these relatives and relate little stories about our own life. We say, "You remember them, don't you?" We say, "Margie says hello." We say, "We love you, and we'll be back soon."

I think when you deliver a loved one to a place like this, you must have the will to block out things. You must have the will to step back and look at the big picture and see that, overall, she is safe here. She will not leave the oven on and burn down her house; she will not walk away from her home and never find her way back. She will be fed and clothed and washed, and if she so much as sneezes, someone will be there to see that she is made well. This is the bright side of La Paloma Blanca.

After a little time passes, it is easier to recall the scent of urine, lurking just under the sharper, piney scent of disinfectant. I think about the aides pushing hampers filled with soiled sheets through the hall. I wonder what it is like to fall asleep and wake up in a place filled with strangers. Confronted with the same situation, I might begin to hit people, too.

Though she has forgotten that I am her grand-daughter, I am still a familiar presence, and so when I visit, Grandma greets me with a smile. One day I find her sleeping in a chair near the nurse's station. I kneel next to her and tap her gently on the shoulder. She stirs a little and then sits up straight. I adjust her glasses and take her hands in my own.

"Hi," I say.

"Hi, yourself," she returns.

She stands, all business, and walks to a large, red metal file cabinet.

"You hungry?" she asks.

"Not really."

"Well, let's see what we've got in the icebox."

She pulls on the drawers of the cabinet, but they don't open. The cabinet is locked.

"Something's wrong," she says. "It's broke or something."

"You know," I say, "I meant to call the guy about that. We'll have to get it fixed. What do you say we take a walk and see if we can find something to eat?"

"Sure," she says. "Maybe that place across town."

"Which place?"

"You know the one."

"I do," I say, and I take her arm and we walk down the hall together.

As we walk, she nods at the nurses and other residents. We pass a man in a wheelchair, and Grandma slows for a minute. Her face softens and her eyes grow bright. She takes my elbow and leans in con-spiratorially. "He was there again last night when I got home."

"Who?" I ask.

"Him. Even though I told him when I left that I'd be mad as hell if I ever saw him again."

"And he was still there?"

"Yep. Plain as day. Sitting out on the lawn."

She's trying to hide a smile. Gran is clearly pleased as hell that this mystery man showed up. She'd maybe even hoped for it. I wonder if she's remembering my grandfather. I know they waited four years before they got married—plenty of time for a few good fights. Did they argue about sex or money or family?

"Was it Everett?" I ask. "Was Grandpa there on the lawn?"

She ignores my question and walks on. I let it drop. Because her speech these days is peppered with pronouns and her mind is playing fast and loose with the structure of time, it's hard to give a solid identity to folks known simply as "she," "he," "her," and "him." Alzheimer's disease is a little like a slot machine. You pull the handle and, with a little luck, sometimes things line up. When they do, it's hard for me not to play along. In today's jackpot, file cabinets are refrigerators, the halls have become streets, and

Gran is nineteen again and playing at being a heart-breaker in her old hometown.

On another visit, I bring my father, and the three of us sit in the common room and watch a cage of finches chatter and hop from branch to branch.

"What do you think of those birds?" I ask, but Grandma is silent.

She takes the fabric of my coat sleeve between her fingers and examines it. "That's a real nice fabric. What kind of fabric is that?"

"It's velvet," I say.

"Well, whatever it is, it sure is nice."

Dad sighs heavily, slides his sleeve up, looks at his wrist, and says, "We should hit it."

"In a minute," I say.

"It's getting late," he says, tapping his wrist, which is, as ever, free of a watch. He leans over and pats Grandma on the knee. "We've got to get going now, Ma," he says.

She looks up at him. "Why didn't little Ross come?" she asks.

"All right, enough's enough," he says. "Let's get the hell out of here."

I kiss Grandma on the head and follow Dad across the room and down the hall and into the clean, clear air outside.

When we reach the car, Dad stops and stares at me hard. "Can you believe that? Little Ross? I'm Ross. She doesn't get it. I'm never coming back to this hellhole."

"You don't have to if you don't want to," I say.

"Is this our car?" Dad asks.

"Sure is," I say.

I unlock his door and help him in, reaching across to fasten his seatbelt. Things like latches and seatbelt fasteners have begun to baffle him, so it's easier if I do it quickly before he gets frustrated. All the while, I'm wondering if it was a good idea to bring him here today. Though we all try to talk around it, we know that Grandma's stint in La Paloma Blanca is a kind of dress rehearsal for what we will encounter with Dad. The things we learn from Gran about Alzheimer's, we will, in the very near future, turn around and apply to her son. When I think about this for too long, I get a tight fluttery feeling in my chest, as though there were a bird trapped in the little cage made by my ribs.

I unlock my own door and climb in beside Dad. He's rummaged around in the glove compartment and found a pen and a few napkins. Using his knee as a table, he hunches over a napkin, sketching out a scene. With a few strokes of his pen, the desert sky stretches vast and endless over a narrow highway curving briefly over the sand before becoming lost in the horizon.

Drawing like this on little scraps of paper is something Dad has always done. When there wasn't a scrap of paper handy, he's been known to draw on the walls of our house. His brain has always seemed to be filled with images longing to take flight. Grandma grew to womanhood cautious to the core, yet that sturdy conviction has been eroded by the winds of Alzheimer's. I wonder how long it will be until Dad's urge to create vanishes. I am grateful for his creativity, for the paintings and drawings he will leave behind. He has made a map of his life, charting out the time before and after my birth and leaving me a history to explore and retrace when he no longer remembers my name. This thought quiets the wings in my chest, at least for now. I give an extra tug on Dad's seatbelt, making sure he's safe before I turn our little car to face the road ahead.

—*Tanya Ward Goodman*

Good Medicine

My eighty-year-old mother leans close to me and whispers, "I'm not sure why, but I can't get something out of my head. Can you help me with it?"

Lately, Mom often "gets stuck" on a specific thought. Her memory and cognitive skills are diminishing. We're not sure if she has Alzheimer's or a form of dementia commonly associated with the Parkinson's disease we know she has. Whatever the cause, repetition in conversation is the norm these days.

For example, when my mother and I leave the assisted-living apartment she shares with my dad, she asks, "Do you have the keys?" I assure her I do. Within less than a minute, she again queries, "Do you have the keys?" Again, I assure her I have them, and I hold them up for her to see. Thirty seconds later she asks, "Do you have the keys?" Frustration punctuates my next response, "Yes! For the third time, I have them!" Her face, too, reflects frustration. Sometimes she wonders why I am so impatient with her; at other times she seems to realize the toll her disease is taking on her mind. Either way, she is dismayed.

Now, here we are again. She's stuck on a thought, and I'm ready to repeat myself over and over and over again. I'm not looking forward to it, but I vow to extend every ounce of patience, kindness, and understanding left in my dwindling reserve to do what I can to comfort her. It's the least I can do, given the seriousness of the situation we are in.

This is the second time in three days that my mother and I are sitting at my father's bedside in the emergency room. He suffers from emphysema and is going through a spell of back-to-back episodes in which he feels he is suffocating and cannot get his breath. His stomach muscles heave as his entire torso works to expand and contract his lungs. His blood pressure is abnormally high. His pulse is racing. He has just commented that it's "time for nature to take its course." He says he can't go on living this way.

An elderly lady in the bed on the other side of the privacy curtain is explaining to the doctor that she has had the flu for four days and can no longer "make water." The curtain-defined exam rooms on a nearby section of the ER contain a young man complaining of numbness in his left arm, a wailing toddler, and a college-age girl describing severe abdominal pains to the attending nurse between moans and cries of "Please make it stop!"

Whatever thought my mother is trying to reconcile or express must certainly be a serious one to distract her from all of that. I reach over and caress her hand in mine. "What's bothering you, Mom? I'll help you."

She leans closer and says, "I just have to know how this ends."

"How what ends, Mother?"

"'Hey diddle diddle, the cat and the . . .'" She pauses, tilts her head to one side, and looks at me with a distant stare.

She can't be serious, I think. *We're in the midst of life-and-death situations, and she's pondering how a childhood nursery rhyme ends?*

I shrink back slightly as I realize she is, indeed, very serious. Her face emanates a naive innocence. Her mind has once again slipped into a childlike state.

"'Fiddle . . . ,'" I gently reply. "'. . . The cow jumped over the moon.'"

She chimes in, "'The little . . .'"

After another pause, I interject, "'Dog . . .'"

"'. . . laughed . . .'" She smiles. "'. . . to see such sport. And the dish ran away with the . . .'"

I return her smile. "'Spoon.' And that's how it ends."

Mom's blue eyes sparkle. "Yes. I knew it. That's how it ends." She pulls her hand free from mine and settles back in the metal folding chair by Dad's bedside, obviously content to have finished the riddle. She closes her eyes, lowers her head, and appears to be resting. We have been in the ER for four hours, and seldom does she last that long without a brief nap.

Dad is also resting easier now. The line displayed on the machine monitoring his breathing shows evenly spaced peaks and valleys. His blood pressure reading is within normal limits. His chest rises and falls with less effort.

On the other side of the curtain, the nurse bumps an IV pole, and it tips over onto a metal table next to the dehydrated flu patient. Dad flinches but resumes a restful state on the edge of deep sleep. Mom jerks, lifts her head, opens her eyes wide, and turns to me.

"'The cow jumped over . . . what?" she puzzles again.

"'The moon,' Mom, 'the moon.'"

Together we get the cat fiddling, the cow jumping, the dog laughing, and the dish running away with the spoon again, not just one more time but several times. Then Mom pulls the warm blanket the ER nurse brought her around her shoulders and lowers her head for another short nap.

I'm left trying to sort out my feelings about what just occurred. I'm worried about my father's health and saddened by my mother's more frequent lapses into her own world, where she is more like a child than the proud and capable mother she once was. I'm tired. I'm frustrated. And still, there is a part of me that can't help but smile and fight the urge to laugh out loud.

A familiar proverb avows that a merry heart promotes healing; and in this instance, God graciously redirected my mother's mind from facing the possibility of her husband's death to the simplicity of a familiar children's rhyme. Her heart was in need of some merriment, and so was mine. We may have been in the shadow of death in that little emergency center, but for at least a while, we feared no evil. Dad was stable. Mom was peaceful. I was reassured of God's presence. Youthful reflection trumped the reality of aging. And a little merriment did our hearts a whole lot of good.

—*Valerie Kay Gwin*

With a Spring in Her Step

The soft, deliberate tap of high-heeled shoes reverberated off the hallway walls outside Dad's hospital room. He looked over at me from his bed, a bit puzzled. We'd enjoyed one another's company for nearly an hour, all the while listening to only the soft squeak-swish-squeak of rubber-soled shoes entering and leaving his room. But the persistent tapping became more forceful and paused outside his door.

Then—like Cinderella sweeping into the ballroom—my mother made her grand entrance. With a spring in her step, she carefully angled through the tangled maze of hospital tables, IV bottles, and chairs. Locking eyes with him, she moved purposefully toward her husband of forty-eight years. My brother, sister-in-law, and I stood mesmerized; this was simply a moment for two.

"I dressed up for you!"

Those five simple words, though stated plainly, spoke volumes: *Together, as a couple, in down-to-earth trust, they would continue to build one another up, to move ahead, and to hold fast to today. For as far as they could see, neither of them would journey through life alone. They could face anything—together. Come hell or high water, they could and would make it.* No statement of faith regarding the unknowns of a vague future was ever made with greater emphasis than with those uncomplicated words of confident assurance.

Life has not been easy the past several years. First, we'd noticed Mother losing her keys more than just a few times. Then it seemed that she would insist on ordering pizza or fried chicken when the family came home, rather than cooking. Having formerly prided herself on being able to time six hot dishes so that all were ready to eat at 5:30 sharp, we were all puzzled when real cooking was relegated only to Christmas.

Next, we started seeing cupboards that were nearly bare and a refrigerator stocked mainly with juice and ancient-looking condiments. Not long after that, we noticed Dad began losing lots of weight. Dad had never cooked more than scrambled eggs, so even though we didn't "get it" at first, eventually things began lining up. The ordinary details of daily living were now slipping from her memory. My brother and

I hastened to move them to an apartment for seniors that would provide a noon meal. Later, Mother confessed that cooking had become overwhelming.

We chose to move them back to the area where they had first set up housekeeping. Both adjusted quickly to apartment living. They enjoyed making connections with new friends in the building and linked up with some people in this town where they'd lived so many years before. Though retired for many years, Dad found a part-time job assisting a farmer with milking cows. Mother began playing the piano for residents in the common room. True, she had now given up doing the checkbook and keeping track of the calendar, but she somehow managed. Life was different, but good.

Their lives together moved along quite healthily as Mother continued on her Alzheimer's meds and Dad regularly visited the cardiologist. Her pace slowed a bit, and he gained a new appreciation for completing jigsaw puzzles. Eventually, they didn't venture out much without my brother or me providing an invitation and transportation. My mother's formerly impeccable outfits gave way to mismatched socks and well drizzled-upon blouses.

Then, one day when Dad's chest tightness became persistent, he was admitted to the large medical center some thirty miles away. His unanticipated admission was surely grounds for great concern. Once he'd settled in, Mother insisted that my brother drive her over to see him. Because none of us anticipated he'd be there long, it seemed ridiculous to attempt to take her for such an exhausting visit. A long ride, tough parking situations, and long hallways would make it a draining day for her physically. We rationalized that in her current state of semi-confusion, she wouldn't really understand why he was there.

But her doggedness prevailed, and my brother finally agreed to pick her up for the journey. To his surprise, he found her neatly attired—heels and all—in the dress Dad had helped her select a few years before. Their shopping together had been a rarity, so we all knew "the dress" was his favorite. After all, he'd hand-selected it. Bright in color, with pleats and flowers, it truly was a sight to behold. And as he knew, when wanting to look her best, Mother would always wear a dress.

My brother and I recall many years before, when Sunday mornings found Mother rising early to fix oatmeal for the family. Before any of us crept out of bed, she would bathe and get partially ready to go to church—for as she put it, "you're not half-dressed until you put on your hose." Then, bustling about in her duster, slippers, and panty hose, she'd make sure the rest of us were ready to go before she'd slip into a dress at the last minute.

As Alzheimer's disease took more of a toll, Mother had given up actually dressing up for church or other community events. None of us had seen her in this Cinderella outfit in years. In fact, my brother and I both would have laid money on the fact that she wouldn't have recognized its significance any longer. Most certainly she would not realize how to match it with her smart, navy patent leather heels. So when my brother had arrived to take Mother to the hospital, he was stunned to find her dressed in all her glory.

At my brother's persistence, she'd finally agreed to switch to comfortable oxford shoes prior to leaving the apartment—but only if he or my sister-in-law would carry the heels that matched her outfit. Therefore, upon their arrival down the hall from Dad's room, a quick shoe swap had occurred, with the comfortable oxfords then hidden quickly behind the curtain at the door.

As Mother made her grand entrance in all of her finery, she immediately heard her sweetheart's low wolf whistle, which she fully expected. She paraded in to show him she could be just like the gal he married—young, pretty, and cheerful! The joy of seeing her light up my Dad's eyes indeed gave me pause. Some corner of her memory came back to life for that special moment.

What a shock the scene was to the rest of us. It was like leaving the door open and finding someone in your household who had gone away and suddenly returned ... but just for this moment. The mother we remembered sashayed back into our lives, if only for a few minutes, to assure Dad that her heart's desire was to always be there to support and encourage him—even in the midst of life's deep unknowns.

—*Yvonne Riege*

It Isn't the End of the World

I remember being a little girl falling down on the pavement and scraping my knee. Although it was a minor hurt, at such a young age it seemed major to me. I began to cry, and when I was certain I had my mother's complete attention, I cried even harder. I will never forget how much better it felt when Mama washed my knee and applied medication and a bandage. She kissed my cheek, held me close, and whispered, "Honey, I know how much it hurts, but believe me, it's not the end of the world."

Years later, when I got engaged to be married, my mother tried to encourage me to take my time and to make certain I had found the right person for a lifetime partner. Head over heels in love, I chose to ignore my mother's warnings. After all, what could a mother know about such things? Later, when my significant other turned out to be a real rat, my heart was crushed. I didn't think I could possibly go on living. Even though Mom had not approved of the relationship, she never said "I told you so." Instead, she held me close and let me cry. Then, sharing my sadness as only a mother could, she told me, "I truly know how much you are hurting, but believe it or not, this isn't the end of the world."

She was so right. Only a year later I met the wonderful man who would soon become my husband. During the first six years of our marriage, God blessed us with five beautiful children. I had never felt as loved or so happy.

Then, seven years into my nearly perfect life, I was diagnosed with multiple sclerosis. I was devastated and certain my life was over. When Mom came to the hospital to see me, I could see she, too, had been crying. She sat on my bed, and for the longest time, we just held each other, unable to talk. Finally, with tearfilled eyes, Mom took my hand in her own and again repeated those same words "I know this is a difficult time and a terrible thing for all of us to accept. Now, more than ever, we have to put our trust and life in God's hands. It could be worse, you know. As bad as it seems, it isn't the end of the world."

Indeed, it wasn't. I have not only seen my five children grow up, I have also experienced the joy of five beautiful grandchildren. My faithful and loving husband has remained by my side throughout the years. Despite multiple sclerosis, I have been truly blessed, and I have lived a very fulfilling and rewarding life.

Then, a year ago, my mom was diagnosed with Alzheimer's disease. Before she progressed to her present state of helplessness, she had temporary periods of normality. During one of these times, while talking with me, she asked, "Now, what is this disease I have? What's wrong with my head? Please be honest with me."

I did my best to tactfully explain the condition and her expected prognosis. I felt like a traitor, conveying this undesirable life sentence on the woman who had always been there for me. My mother was a very intelligent person, and I can't imagine how painful it must have been for her to be told she had this mind-stripping illness. It broke my heart, and I wanted to run away, but she'd asked for the truth and so I honored her wishes.

Mama listened carefully to my every word and seemed to grasp all that I was saying. When I was done, she remained quiet for a long time, lost in a world of her own, seemingly far away. Then suddenly her eyes met mine. So like my mom, even in the midst of her own private hell, she put my feelings first.

"Now, what are you crying for? I'm the one who is sick this time," she said gently. "You must be brave enough for both of us. Oh God, I know how much this hurts you, but regardless of what happens to me, you've got to be strong. In spite of what you think right now, I promise you, this isn't the end of the world."

Mama was right.

Her disease progressed rapidly. Soon she was no longer able to hold me close and to say all the right things to soothe my pain. In troubled times, she couldn't assure me that all would be well in time, that my world would continue. I so missed her gentle encouragement, but I knew that it was my turn to be the strength in her life. Because she no longer remembered the words, I used mine to repeat the prayers she'd taught me so long ago. I used my ears to listen to her constant meaningless chatter. For a long while, Mama still understood kisses, and returning the ones she'd given me for so many years helped to ease her pain.

On rare occasions, Mama would smile, but most of the time she was extremely depressed. Many of her friends and relatives stopped going to see her because it made them feel uncomfortable. At first that upset me, but then I realized that maybe they were not fortunate enough to have had a sweet, gentle lady telling them that no matter how painful or uncomfortable life gets, it truly isn't the end of the world.

Three days ago, my brother, sister, and I were gathered in my mother's room shortly after she had passed away, crying and wondering how we would go on without our mother. None of us were ready to say good-bye, but we had no choice. As I stood there I was suddenly filled with peace. From a faraway place, I could hear my mother whisper, "Cry for the loss you feel in your heart but also be happy for me, for I am with God in a place that is more wonderful than you can imagine. I am so happy now. Yes, honey, I am gone from your life but never from your heart. For the last time, I promise you, it isn't the end of your world."

I know that my mother was right. I have no doubt that her love and wisdom is with me always, shining light on my darkest hours and bringing joy to all my days.

—*Barbara Jeanne Fisher*

Teaspooned Victories

If I were to describe my grandmother, adjectives like "industrious," "hardworking," and "productive" would come to mind. Born in 1901, she had witnessed two world wars, survived the Great Depression, and managed to provide a college education for her four children by working in a factory. She had accomplished all this years before I made my entrance into this world in 1956. No wonder I had never seen my grandmother idle; she had no time! The few occasions I can remember her seated in the "parlor," she was busy, her workbasket at her side. There were always socks to be darned, skirts to be hemmed, and tablecloths to be mended. Even while relaxing, she worked, often with a rabbit-eared, black-and-white television tuned to a Sunday night program for company.

What an ultimate irony that such an active, productive woman should spend the last years of her life completely idle—first, sitting in a wheelchair; then, lying in a hospital bed . . . initially, confused and frustrated; later, listless and vacant. *Gram, where are you?* I remember silently asking. *What happened to that vibrant, active woman, and who is this shell that had been left behind?*

Now, looking back over the last few months preceding my grandmother's rapid decline, I realize there were harbingers of the devastation to come. Why I had refused to acknowledge them remains a mystery, but back in the late 1960s, Alzheimer's disease was not a commonly used term or diagnosis. It would take another decade to bring this condition to the forefront. Ironically, just as my grandmother and her peers had headed the country's campaign to give women the right to vote in their youth, they had shined the nation's spotlight on the issue of age-related dementia in their twilight years.

My grandmother's descent into that lost world began with what I can only describe as inappropriate reactions to common annoyances. Things like a broken shoelace, a coffee spill, or a traffic jam would become catastrophic. What my grandmother would have usually handled with a shrug or a shake of her head would now evoke a sudden anger, a hostile outburst, and sometimes even tears. That she'd always had a calm and quiet nature made these behaviors even more bizarre.

Additional peculiarities soon followed. One day, for example, she picked up a bunch of bananas that were ripening in her kitchen. Gently, she proceeded to peel every one of them. When she was finished, she stared at the pile of yellow skins and white bananas for hours. Finally, she asked me what they were and how they got that way. Another time, she sat at the kitchen table, where she folded a linen napkin into a tiny perfect square. She stared at it, carefully unfolded it, and then repeated the entire process over and over again for nearly three hours.

While those incidents were disturbing, at least there were tranquil interludes among them, for which I would have been more grateful had I known what was to come. As my grandmother's condition worsened, she became combative, bordering on abusive. One day she emptied her entire closet, and with her dresses, sweaters, and blouses draped over her arm, she announced she was leaving; it was four o'clock in the morning. When we gently attempted to restrain her, she became violent—thrashing, kicking, and demanding to be "let out" of the place she had called home for nearly forty years.

Of course, our family sought medical expertise and professional assistance, but in the 1970s, such services were few and far between. The various diagnoses ranged from "hardening of the arteries," "senility," "acute forgetfulness," and "lack of short-term memory." Those of us who have witnessed the odd behaviors, mood swings, and other devastating affects of Alzheimer's disease on individuals afflicted with it, such descriptions barely scratched the proverbial surface.

Reflecting on the years of my grandmother's "sickness," I wish I could call to mind a blessing of some sort that this condition had wrought. I have read that sometimes caregivers experience a Zen-like state while feeding a loved one, dressing a parent, or assisting a spouse in the simple activities of daily living, or "ADLs" as the professionals refer to such actions. According to many such testimonials, the very disease that consumed the life force of their loved ones with such a vengeance sometimes doled it back in measured teaspoons—a flicker of recognition, a whisper of a long-forgotten name, a trace of a favorite expression. Such small "victories" seemed to fuel these caregivers, providing them with some measure of comfort.

But I found no such solace. I was angry. Why should my dear grandmother, who worked so hard for so many years, be sentenced to ending her life in such a state? Why should a woman who had never known the luxury of leisure be spending her last years in a perverted, wanton state of it—languishing in a wheelchair and a hospital bed? Why should a woman who was so vibrant and so bright, who never drank, smoked, or gambled, be punished so severely? And selfishly, why should I be deprived of the grandmother I had loved? I had no answers.

After battling the disease for a dozen years, my grandmother passed on. Her funeral was almost a relief, as all of us felt the woman we had loved had left us long ago. Her memorial service was a final tribute to a woman her younger grandchildren had never had the privilege of knowing, as I had. Somehow, that "privilege" short-circuited my anger.

Years later, with the gifts of time and distance, I began to view my grandmother's illness with more objectivity, if that was at all possible. And since her passing, I have come to appreciate what I refer to as the "randomness of life." Unfortunately, just as random acts of kindness can bestow blessings to anonymous recipients from unknown donors, the antithesis can also occur: The first-time tourist to New York City who randomly enjoyed an early morning coffee on the observation deck of the World Trade Center on September 11, 2001, but never exits the building. The middle-aged couple from Denver who rang in the 2005 New Year vacationing in the Maldive

Islands and is randomly lost in the tsunami. The child conceived by two healthy parents who randomly receives from each the gene for Huntington's disease.

I have come to realize that, although I cannot control any such tragedy—be it a terrorist attack, a force of nature, a genetic anomaly, or a disease—I can control how I handle it. My grandmother's battle with Alzheimer's disease was no exception.

Looking back, I wish I could have gotten past my own anger at that time. My perception was that somehow this disease was a personal one, a deliberate act against her, our family, and even me. It wasn't. If I could have viewed her condition differently, perhaps I would have recognized and savored those teaspooned victories—the flickers of recognition, the whispers of a long-forgotten name, and the traces of a favorite expression. I wish I had.

—*Barbara Davey*

Going Home

Monday evening she heard him rummaging through the bathroom again. She called down the hall, "Carl, what are you doing?"

"Packing," he hollered.

Shaking her head, Marilyn went back to the kitchen to start dinner. Carl had it in his head for quite a while that they had to leave their home of many years and find their "real" house. *Maybe he just misses our old home,* Marilyn speculated. *That could be why he keeps packing the car full of his things and saying we have to find that other house.*

Marilyn picked up the carrot peeler and began scraping the skin off a carrot while she thought. *No, that can't be it. We've lived here in the country a long time, and he's loved every minute of it. After we moved, he told me again and again how great it was to live here.*

Her lip trembled as her hand stopped scraping. *I won't*, she told herself fiercely. *I won't let it get to me.*

Then she heard a crash in the bathroom and shouted, "Carl, what was that?"

"Nothing—just dropped a can of hairspray," he yelled back.

She sighed and went back to cooking while she ruminated. *No. I think he realizes that, even though he doesn't remember he has Alzheimer's, something is wrong. He wants to go back, to a time when life was good, a place that doesn't make him feel anxious and confused. If only I could help him.*

Carl walked past her with a bulging sports bag and a pillow. "You coming?" he asked.

"Not right now, Carl. We have to eat dinner first. Then we can go."

A pang of guilt pierced her. The support group had told her to just agree with him and pretend to go along, and later he would forget. They were right, too. It worked every night, and she could unpack the car after he went to bed. But it felt so wrong, so much like lying. Why couldn't she just reason with him and get him to see this was their home? With a sigh, she finished scraping one carrot and started on another. It was going to be a long week.

Then she thought, *Hey, maybe we can go on a vacation! I'd have to get some things done in advance, but it could be done.*

As they ate their dinner, she brought it up. "Carl, would you like to go to the Oregon Coast? We could relax, read books, and walk on the beach. What do you think?"

He twirled his spoon in the stew and looked up at her. He still had those piercing blue eyes that were impossible to read. As he lifted the spoon to his mouth he said, "Could we look for our real house on the way?"

She sighed. "Maybe we could do that on the way home."

Friday morning, Marilyn woke Carl early. "I need you to help me in the garden today, honey. We have to get it mulched and watered really well, because we're going to the Oregon Coast for a week, remember?"

"Okay. Can I pack now?" he asked.

"After we get the garden done. Then we'll both pack."

She cooked oatmeal while Carl took a shower. *This might be just what we need,* she reflected. *Yes, just like so long ago when we went on our honeymoon and he sang love songs to me on the beach. What a wonderful time it was. Maybe this will bring some of him back to me again.*

After breakfast, they worked in the garden. Carl was like his old self, shoveling and working as hard as two men. He didn't mention looking for the house or any of the other strange dreams he had that were so real to him when he repeated them out loud.

"Marilyn, remember when we first bought this place? It took so long to get those pipe lines dug from the well up to the house."

"Yes, and remember how the kids complained when we made them help?" she said. "You'd think we'd forced them to be our slaves all their lives instead of asking them to do two or three hours of work to help get the ditch started."

He chuckled and nodded. "Those kids, they were pretty soft when we bought this place. Nothing like hard work to bring out character in a person."

He spoke so normally that she began to sink into that feeling that everything was going to be the way it used to be when he took care of the bills, the broken household appliances, and the problems, before things began spinning out of control.

"Well, looks like we're done here. Let's go pack now, Carl."

"Time to find our real house, right?"

Her smile faded. "Okay, let's find our real home, Carl."

They packed and got ready, but then she had to look for an hour to find the keys Carl had moved to a "better" spot so they wouldn't get lost. Finally, when she was just about to give up, there they were.

"Under your hat on the hood of the car is a 'better' spot?" she scolded.

He muttered something and stared at her. There were those blue eyes again—piercing through her spirit and penetrating her heart, asking her to forgive him, not to blame him, to remember what was wrong, not to be angry.

She repented and said, "Oh, let's go. We need to get to Julie's by five."

Carl obediently got in and buckled up. "Julie who?" he asked.

"Julie, our daughter," she stressed. He couldn't forget that—not yet!

As she drove, he fell asleep and she murmured a prayer. *Let me have some grace, please? I know I need to change the way I think about him, but I just don't know how to do it after fifty years of his being in charge.*

Carl woke up for a minute and said, "Hey, that sign says fifty-five miles per hour. How fast are you going, Marilyn?"

Sigh. "Fifty-five."

"Okay. Just wanted to be sure." He fell back asleep.

When they reached Julie's place, Carl was tired and cranky. He'd slept most of the way, but he needed another nap because traveling stressed him out. Marilyn visited with Julie and helped prepare dinner while he slept.

"He keeps saying he wants to find our real house," she said. "I'm so tired of it!"

"Well, at least he doesn't fight with you a lot or get mad and break things. Maybe thinking about positive things like that would help."

"Nothing helps when I don't know what to do."

When dinner was almost ready, Carl came into the kitchen. His grandson, Noah, ran up to give him a hug.

"Hi, Dad. How are you doing?" Julie asked.

"I don't know. . . . Were you there when I met your mother?"

She couldn't think of an answer.

He said, "I guess you couldn't have been, could you?" Then he walked over to the sink, reached into his pocket, pulled out a big pile of coins, and began dropping them in the sink.

"Grampa, what're you doing?" Noah asked.

Not answering, Carl began to wash the coins. Noah watched. When his Grampa started drying them off with a paper towel, Noah asked again, "What're you doing?"

Startled, Carl whispered, "I can't talk now. I'm doing a scientific experiment."

Noah watched as he counted the coins into piles of quarters, nickels, dimes, and pennies. Then Carl pulled some baggies out of the drawer and put the coins into separate bags. "These coins," he informed the curious Noah, "are for church. Don't let me forget to bring them." Then he put the bags in his pocket and sat at the table.

Dinner conversation was normal, except that Carl told the story about walking through the snowy woods to find firewood when he was a kid several times. Julie pulled her mother aside as they got ready for bed.

"Mom, are you sure you'll be all right driving another four hours to Oregon?"

"Yes, I drive with him all the time. He usually just sleeps or reads me the signs and tells me how to drive."

Julie looked worried, but said, "I guess you know what you're doing."

The next morning they left early. After everyone hugged good-bye, Marilyn got into the driver's seat again. Carl smiled at her as he sat down in the front passenger seat. "Are we going to the ocean now?" he asked.

Startled that he remembered, she said, "Well, yes! We'll be there in four hours."

He leaned back. As she started off, he began to sing "In the Misty Moonlight," where anywhere was alright "as long as I'm with yoooooou."

As they drove, Carl serenaded her with song after song, remembering each one perfectly, just as he had sung them so many years before on the beach. He even sang her favorite, "Melody of Love." Marilyn's smile glowed like the bonfire on the beach at night. He still loved her, just like when they went on their honeymoon so long ago.

He stopped singing for a minute and read a road sign, "Fifty miles to Seaside, Oregon. Is that where we're going?"

"Yes, dear."

Carl closed his eyes and started another song, singing with joyful abandon and with longing for the "dear hearts and gentle people" of his "hometown."

Unexpected joy flooded Marilyn's heart. She knew where his real home was, after all. They would find it in their hearts when they comforted each other through these hard times. *Thank you,* she prayed, glancing upward. *I know it still won't be easy, but at least now I know how to give him what his spirit needs.*

Carl stopped singing and asked, "Can we still look for our real house on the way home, my sweet bride?"

"Of course we can. We'll watch for it on the way there, too, honey," she answered.

—Suzanne Endres

To Be Present

The phone rang as I closed the oven door on a well-stuffed turkey. It was Dad. He should have been circling nearby on an incoming flight on this Thanksgiving day; instead, he was calling from Texas.

"Texas?" I yelped before regaining my calm to hear him explain some impossible sequence of events that had resulted in him flying to the wrong state.

These kinds of fantastic events were happening to Dad more and more frequently—like the time he drove us down the left side of the street for two blocks while insisting that it was the fault of poor signage. Only after I insisted for the third time that no matter what was causing him to drive into oncoming traffic, it would be infinitely safer for him to return to the correct side of the road, did he oblige.

Shortly after that drive, the tests began. He protested; I insisted. Can't say I blame him. What accomplished seventy-one-year-old man wants to be bossed around by his twenty-three-year-old daughter, especially on matters that might result in devastating news. Doctors confirmed what I'd been losing sleep about. Dementia, later diagnosed as Alzheimer's, was pulling the cognitive carpet out from under my dear father's feet.

Even after the medical writing was on the wall, deciding how to plan for this sadly unacceptable and degenerative process was excruciating. Overnight, I was shoved into an unfamiliar role—before, I had always been his child; now, I would become his keeper, his guardian, and his mother. Dad and I listened as the doctors stoically announced that he shouldn't be driving or working or living alone. They encouraged him to move 3,000 miles to live near me so he "could be taken care of." We walked out of the neatly carpeted medical office and blinked blindly into the Miami sun. We stood, lost in a new reality and dazed by all we'd been flatly told, and silently wondered how to proceed. Finally, Dad unlocked the passenger door for me and then climbed into the driver's seat.

We sat for a moment before I began, "Dad, the doctors said you shouldn't..."

"Let's talk about it at dinner," he interjected. It was too much, too fast, too overwhelming.

"Okay," I relented. "But please drive on the right side of the road because I could really use a drink."

Over a pitcher of sake and tuna rolls, Dad and I uncomfortably discussed what we'd been told only an hour before. I told him I wanted to support him in making decisions now, while he was still able to make decisions, about things like where he wanted to live and how to bow out of his fifty-year career. By the time dessert arrived, his eyes were glazed over. He couldn't process any more.

The next morning I pushed onward, broaching one beastly subject after another over a steamy plate of eggs benedict and potent coffee, until his face, once again, went blank. Dad didn't know what he wanted to do. He didn't want to change anything, let alone everything that mattered to him. He wasn't ready to give up his independent life and all the things that gave it meaning and defined who he was. And I wasn't ready to take it all away from him, either. As we waited for the cab to take me to the airport, we sidestepped our paralysis by agreeing to keep talking in hopes of making a definitive plan by the end of the month.

Weeks turned into another month, and then the phone call came. Apparently, I had waited too long to usurp my dad's independence. Confused about the time of day, he'd given himself repeated doses of insulin and then driven to work. The car was crushed on both sides and covered with mud and foliage. His death-defying adventure brought him into the yard of a thankfully kindhearted woman. She helped him out of the car and, unable to decipher what he was saying, called the number on his business card. He wound up in a coma, and I boarded a plane to be by his bedside.

After Dad came out of intensive care, I flew him back with me to Seattle. Mid-flight, he thanked me for coming, put on his hat, picked up his brief-case, smoothed out his trench coat, stood up, and announced he needed to get on the road to his next meeting and would be in touch. When I explained that we were on an airplane and there was no place to go until we landed, he smiled and said, "Of course, I'll do some work." Then he rifled through his brief-case before thanking me for coming, smoothing his trench coat, and standing to repeat the whole thing again.

We went through this routine several more times before he became angry and impatient with me. "Jenny, I really need to go. This isn't funny."

I reached under my tray to discreetly extract and pulverize the little pink sedative the doctor had given me in case this kind of thing were to happen. Into his orange juice it went. "Please, try this fresh juice before rushing off to your meeting," I connived, giving him a sip. As I watched sleep overtake him, I imagined the shocking news headline of our day: *Daughter drugs her own father.*

As the months passed and my father's mind slowly dissolved, I marveled at how his mannerisms, values, and habits stayed relatively intact. Only the substance was evaporating, leaving enough of his essence to remind me of who he used to be. Every thoughtful rub of his chin, each request for the morning paper, and the daily donning of his blazer, Greek captain's hat, and trench coat all created the appearance of the man I'd always known. It was immensely comforting.

Though Alzheimer's relentlessly eroded his intellect, filched his short-term memory, and interrupted his independence, it generously left his inveterate sense of humor, his entrenched kindness, his trademark habits, and the beguiling sparkle in his eyes. I had such a conflicted relationship with this disease, often feeling both an angry "screw you, Alzheimer's, for what you are taking away" and a simultaneous "thank you, Alzheimer's, for what you have left behind."

Several times a week I would pick up my dad from the nursing home and take him to a café. It was one of his favorite things. We'd get a paper, order him a latte, and sit together at the wobbly round table next to the window. After two loud sips of coffee, he would ceremoniously open the first section of the paper, then with legs crossed and glasses moved to the tip of his nose, he would begin his rhythmic slurps of caffeinated pleasure over his morning newspaper. This scene, if viewed through a wide-angle lens, could be one from ten, twenty, even forty years before. This fantasy, however, was discredited by one new detail that was visible only to the discerning eye: Dad was "reading" the newspaper upside down.

Just when I would get lulled into accepting the fairly steady march of Dad's dementia and the pervasive confusion of his mind, we would stumble into a rare moment of pristine clarity. The clouds would clear and there would be my dad . . . as if we had washed up on the shores of a sandy island of an unchanged yesteryear, surrounded but untouched by the lapping waves of the sea of our Alzheimer's reality. We could stay only an instant before the ground evaporated under our grateful souls and left us swimming in an ocean of Alzheimer's once again.

I remember one such clearing of the clouds when Dad was in the hospital after a bad fall that left him with a nasty gash on his head and more confused than usual. For hours, he talked intermittently, eyes closed, in a secret language for which I lacked a decoder. I listened intently, hoping to grasp some shred of meaning in his nonsensical sentences. Discouraged and exhausted, I let my mind wander for a second. My eyes fell on his parched lips. *He must be thirsty,* I thought, and rose to fill a Dixie cup with water from the hospital basin. I put the cup to his lips, and he drank tiny sip after tiny sip.

Suddenly, he grabbed my hand in his, opened his eyes and locked them on mine, and said, "You are such a good daughter. Thank you."

I froze in shock and joy, hoping that if I didn't move or breathe he would get to stay this way, here with me, intact, alert, and aware. Maybe the whole thing had been a mistake or a trick. Perhaps he'd just been lost and now he was back, free to return to his regular life, and we could reclaim our old identities, me as his daughter and he as my father. As quickly as they'd left, the clouds returned, and Dad closed his eyes as the secret language spilled out again. He was gone. But where did he go? Was he in there somewhere? Like all the times before, I grew weary of these unanswerable questions and instead chose to replay that delicious, fleeting moment of clarity and connection over and over in my mind, basking in the nourishment of his little visit, eternally thankful for what felt like a rare drink of water in a vast desert.

Oh my, were there hilarious times under the spell of Alzheimer's. For example, I arrived at the nursing home one day to attend Dad's care conference and was greeted by him at the door. He was ready, briefcase in hand, business face on, and two neatly pressed and knotted ties snug at his neck atop a lavender turtleneck that must have lost its formerly white self after taking one too many spins with a dark load of laundry. I suppressed my surprise, horror, and laughter all at the same time to walk with him to the conference room. I decided against saying anything to Dad about his unprecedented fashion statement, certain he had no idea what he was wearing. We sat at the shiny conference table waiting for the staff to arrive.

Dad must have caught me staring at him, because he said, through a mischievous grin, "You like my outfit? Two ties are all the rage—I'm cutting edge."

A fan of Houdini and a practitioner of magic himself, my dad took pride in his crafty escapes from the nursing home. He was so successful that the facility had to paint exit doors with elaborate murals of garden walls, install alarms, and issue electronic bracelets to residents just to slow him down. Undeterred, Dad hatched a new strategy based on the medication-dispensing schedule of the staff. He watched their routines and knew when they would be occupied at the other end of the building for a certain number of minutes. He secretly shared his plan with all residents in his wing who were even slightly mobile. When the time was right, he set his plan into motion, gathering up his neighbors and clustering them around the patio door. Once everyone was in place, he waited for the nurse to head down the hall with her medication cart before he gave the signal and pushed open the double doors. Alarms blaring, Dad and his jailbreak crew hustled in their weary, wobbly, walker-assisted ways out into the blossoming garden patio. Though they didn't get far before the staff came running, Dad and his team were gleeful over their victorious moments in the sun.

Dad's neighbor and only male peer in the nursing home was a sweet, tall man named Forest. My dad and Forest would wander back and forth into each other's rooms all day, going through each other's drawers and closets, putting on mismatched socks, and losing various sweaters and hats. One day Forest walked into Dad's room, as he often did while I was visiting, and once there looked unsure of why he'd come.

"Hello, Forest. How's your day going?" I asked.

Forest thought for a moment before answering in a matter-of-fact tone, "Well, sometimes I have days, but today isn't one."

It made beautiful sense.

What a gift it was to be able to love, laugh, weep, witness, and respect my dad through his ride with Alzheimer's. As excruciating as it was to watch him slip away, I am thankful that I resisted the urge to distance myself in an effort to somehow avoid his painful reality. To be present in relation to the raw vulnerability that the disease created felt like a sacred act. As he took his last breaths, I told him it was okay to let go, if it felt like it was time. I felt the openness of a good-bye unfettered by any stockpile of regret, and I knew I had done right by him.

—Jenoa Briar-Bonpane

Tell Me Not to Worry

I am sitting at my jumbled desk working on an essay when the phone rings. The joy in my cousin Lenore's voice pulses over the line from her home in Ohio to mine in Oregon. She's had two of her own poems and several of her translations of Chinese classical poetry accepted by an excellent "little magazine."

"Lenore," I say, "that's so great. You've escaped."

"So far," she says.

Lenore is in her mid-eighties and still razor sharp, so there's a good chance she's evaded Alzheimer's, the terrible disease that stole the minds and lives of both her mother and our grandmother. According to some studies, people with one first-degree rela-tive—a parent or a sibling—are 3.5 times more likely to develop the disease than the rest of the popula-tion. In our conversations over the years, Lenore has often talked of her fear of becoming part of those statistics.

My mother, Lenore's aunt, escaped Alzheimer's, too. She was eighty-eight and still writing and teaching classes about writing when she had a massive stroke. Her mother was not so fortunate.

Grandma was confused and afraid most of the time that she lived with my family, off and on, as I was growing up. I can picture her still, silver hair always in a tight bun at the back of her neck, frail body always in a blue dress of some soft fabric. A grandmother might not be a first-degree relative, but it's a close brush with this dreaded disease that literally causes your brain to die cell by cell. I can't think of anything more terrifying than literally losing my mind. So now that I've turned the big six-oh, I'm on a daily Alzheimer's alert.

About the time I finish chatting on the phone with Lenore, my husband, Ray, wanders into my office. "Look at this red thing on my leg," he says, pointing to what looks like either a mosquito or a spider bite. Once upon a time Ray and I misdiagnosed shingles, thinking a raised red spot on his chest was an insect bite, so I understand his concern. But he isn't sick today, as he was then, and I'm confident there's no need to worry.

"Just put some of that . . . that . . . that pink stuff on it," I say.

Damn. I can picture the bottle in the medicine cabinet. It's pink, as is the thick liquid inside. But even if somebody paid me a million dollars to remember its name right now, I couldn't.

I'm forever questioning the meaning of incidents like this. Although "senior moments" are so common among the over-fifty population that they are the subject of numerous e-mail attachments circulating around the country, if not the world, it's easy to confuse them with indications of the early onset of Alzheimer's. I keep an article beside my bed that has a chart showing the signs of normal aging versus the warning signs of Alzheimer's. According to the chart, in normal aging you forget a word but it comes to you later. Three hours after Ray asked me to check the bite on his leg, when I'm out in the garden fighting blackberries, the words "Calamine Lotion" come to me. Phew. Just a senior moment. Safe so far.

Ray lost his mother to Alzheimer's a little more than a year ago. His aunt and grandfather died of it, too. He's one of those three-times-as-likely statistics, so he's even more nervous than I. He returns to the garden now, a big patch of pink where the bite is.

"Do you know where my keys are?" he asks, close to panic. "I can't find them anywhere. I never used to lose my keys."

Actually, he's lost them several times a week for as long as I've known him. He has four sets, and when they all disappear he goes on an exhaustive key hunt through pants pockets, under car mats, among miscellaneous magazines and decks of playing cards. But I don't laugh at his panic. Alzheimer's isn't a laughing matter.

"Remember the chart," I tell him. "Temporarily misplacing your keys is normal. Forgetting the purpose of a key would be a problem."

"I know the purpose of a key." Ray's voice has that trace of irritation it gets when I sound like the teacher I was for many years. "We're going to need one if we're going to be at the Jensen's on time."

I look at my watch. Wow, the time on this lovely summer afternoon has passed quickly. I put away my clippers and take a quick shower. Ray finds a set of keys in his bicycling jacket, and we head out.

I'm chatting away about nothing much when I suddenly notice that the residential neighborhood we're driving through doesn't look familiar. We've been to the Jensen's half a dozen times. They live in a well-established area with lots of foliage, and these streets are lined with newer homes and young trees.

"Do you know where we are?" I ask.

"Come to think of it, this doesn't look right, does it?"

I can't criticize Ray. I haven't been paying atten-tion, and besides, I, too, get easily lost when driving.

"I was so sure I knew the way," Ray says. "Maybe I'm getting Alzheimer's."

Confusion about directions is a common sign of Alzheimer's, but we have both been navigationally challenged our whole lives, so to be in this strange neighborhood without a clue which way to turn is more annoying than worrisome. We are capable of turning the wrong way with a map right under our nose. Being lost on the way to the Jensen's doesn't even rate as a senior moment. It's the way Ray and I do life.

"There's a major road down there," I say. "Either it will look familiar, or we can ask someone."

We reorient ourselves successfully, arrive at the Jensen's only a few minutes late, feast on a delicious salmon dinner, and then look at photos of a hiking trip we recently took together. When we get home after a delightful evening, I have just one thing left on my to-do list for the day. I wrote a big check for our house insurance, and now I want to make sure it has cleared with enough left in the house account to cover the mortgage payment going through tomor-row on auto-pay.

Within moments I'm staring at the computer screen, alarm bells ringing in my head. *What have I done?* I see that a check to State Farm has cleared, but the amount of the check is two hundred dollars, not close to a thousand as it should have been. *Did I get two bills from the insurance company, one for two hundred dollars and then the bigger homeowner's insurance premium that hasn't cleared yet? Maybe some little add-on for our umbrella policy that I've forgotten?*

I click on "detail" and bring up an enlargement of the front of the check. There it is. State Farm. $200.00. Check #200.

No. Tell me I didn't write the check number instead of the amount on the bill. That ranks as major confusion. Maybe even Alzheimer's confusion.

I tell myself that if I did have Alzheimer's, I wouldn't be able to figure out my mistake, but it still takes hours to get to sleep. My mind does scary things, like plan the affairs I'd better get in order quickly, before I fail even more, and the care Ray will need to line up for me when the disease gets worse.

I wake with a headache that doesn't go away until the insurance office opens and I can call and talk to someone. "Could you please look up my record?" I ask, trying for a calm voice. "I've written a check to you for two hundred dollars, and I'm not sure if I was billed for something of that amount or I made a mistake."

My breath is tight in my chest while the agent looks up the information. "There it is," she says after a long moment. "Looks like a partial payment on your homeowner's premium."

So I did look at the number 200 on the check instead of the invoiced amount. How could I do that if my brain was still intact?

"Don't worry," she says cheerfully. "They'll bill you for the rest."

She can tell me not to worry. Alzheimer's probably doesn't run in *her* family.

Ray comes into my office to find out what's taking me so long and sees me crumpled at my desk, my head on my arms. Embarrassed to tell even him, I explain what happened.

"When did you write the check?" he asks.

I pull out my check register and see that I wrote it the morning we were doing three things simultaneously before we left on a trip to the Coast: catching up on a hundred tasks, such as paying bills, packing the car for the trip, and preparing to host an afternoon baby shower for my daughter-in-law before taking off. We often over-schedule ourselves with physical and mental activities, but even for us, that was multitasking to the max. I suppose doing all those things at once could scramble anyone's mind.

Could the insurance agent be right? Am I worrying too much? Alzheimer's is a terrible disease. A dear friend of mine who headed an Alzheimer's organization here in Portland, when faced with a diagnosis of terminal cancer, said, "As long as I can think, I can stand anything." But I'm devoting a lot of time and energy to worrying about something that may never happen. Even if I'm more likely than some folks to get Alzheimer's, with my busy, active lifestyle, chances are good I won't.

Slow down, I tell myself. *Breathe in. Breathe out.* Several people I know who haven't even experienced their first hot flash have made banking errors. In fact, I made more serious mistakes than this long before I turned sixty and put myself on Alzheimer's alert. The time I forgot to pick up my daughter from kindergarten comes to mind. I can still hear her voice on the school phone when I think about it. "Mommy? Are you coming to get me?"

The agent was right. I need to quit seeing the "A" word every time I make a mistake. It's a lot more fun biking, hiking, reading, writing, going to concerts and plays, and visiting with friends and family than painting dark mental pictures of an unknown future. I'm going off Alzheimer's alert.

—Samantha Ducloux Waltz

Sign Here, Please

As I let myself into the Alzheimer's unit, I felt like an extra-terrestrial passing through an airlock on a spaceship: 1-2-3-4-*, press the handle, shove the hip, I'm in. I wondered again, *Who's the crazy one?*

Shortly after Dad arrived at the nursing home, we needed to move the automatic pension and Social Security payments from the bank in his hometown to the bank in ours. Who knew that the powers of attorney held by both my mother and brother were no good with the federal government? I didn't understand this, despite my Ivy League doctorate, but queerly, I found I could accept that the government had no faith in our legal system. In order for Mom to move the Social Security payment from the old bank account to the new, she was told to appear in person at the so-called "local" Social Security office forty miles away, which was "manned" by an answering machine. We left several messages asking for a call back.

The trouble was that Mom got confused about paperwork. Without my sister or me there to help, she couldn't explain her question well enough to the clerks maintaining the databases at the other end of the phone. And, naturally, the offices would not make an appointment at a certain time to call you back. Of course, they claimed they would do that—or rather, the national hotline said that the local office would do it. In fact, it didn't happen.

As for Dad's pension, the blue chip company sent a simple form for him to fill out and sign. No, Mom couldn't sign for him, despite her power of attorney. Hmm. Neither government nor the private sector would honor a duly executed legal document. This boded ill for what promised to be a legally and financially complicated future. The feeling of insecurity was excruciating. Mom looked at me with pleading eyes; I was used to them by now. But what had I gotten myself into? Was Dad really crazy? Or was I the crazy one? The situation had gone berserk.

Some would have simply forged a signature, but I was my father's daughter—all about following procedures to the letter. So Mom and I had filled out the form, and now I was taking it to my father in the Alzheimer's unit.

I placed the form gingerly in front of Dad and said, "We're moving your pension deposit to the bank out here, Dad, and they need you to sign this paper."

He balked, his forehead wrinkling both horizontally and vertically at once, a facial expression that covered confusion as well as disapproval. He couldn't make sense of it, and it scared him as well. "No," he said, bristling. He pushed the paper away.

I tried again, and again he pushed it away. I slumped back in the plastic-form chair and looked out the window. Through the yard and over the eight-foot-high solid wood fence, I could see only the sky. Gradually, it gave way to a scene from the past, a time two years before, during the spring after Dad had gone into the hospital for his back operation.

That afternoon, I had sat in his den, staring out into a Pennsylvania sky. It had looked exactly the same. Mom hadn't said a thing, just looked at me with her clear child's eyes. She did not want to make medical decisions for Dad, though she clearly understood that someone had to. She had been confused and tongue-tied during the weeks after his operation, repeatedly thanking me for staying with her. Time after time, I had witnessed her deferring to the doctors without asking a single question. Because she had a master's degree in nursing from Yale, I knew her hesitancy was because she was scared. So I had asked Dad to sign a medical power of attorney for one of his children. It felt awkward; he had always made not only his own decisions but also the decisions for the entire family. But it also felt like the right thing to do. Though I appeared to him to be an alien, I hoped I could convince him that I was an alien with a good heart.

He was irate. Sweat burst from his skin like rain from a thundercloud. Even though he was sitting in his desk chair with his back to me, I seemed to be looking up all of his six feet, two inches into his angry face from the height of a five-year old. I steeled myself for a battle I knew I had to win, then I felt myself falter.

He turned toward me but could hardly speak. He mumbled something about "trusting your mother," which trailed off into a shamed look that pleaded, *Please go away. I don't want to talk about this.*

I didn't know what to do next. He didn't want to admit that he didn't trust us, and his fear continued to rain down on me and soak me coldly to my own bones. Finally I said, "Well, think about it," and turned to go.

"I don't need to think about it," he snapped pretty nastily, but I knew he had no choice.

I waited five days before bringing up the subject again. I reminded him that my sister was expert at dealing with the health care system, which she had done professionally for most of her life. I told him I was going to sign one for myself, if she would agree to take on my health care, too. He wouldn't budge. I felt the issue was so important, I finally exploded.

"You're not this stupid!" I yelled at him. "I'm ashamed of you for putting Mom in that position. It isn't fair. If you can't sign it over to one of your own children, then pick somebody else you do trust. I'm sure one of your old friends around here would do it."

He ducked around to face his desk and said nothing. Why didn't he trust his own daughter?

A few days later he had three copies of medical powers of attorney, one with each of his children's names on it. He called me into the den and gave me mine. There was no more discussion. I had won. He felt beaten and diminished, lost now that he had to depend on someone else. He experienced my request for a power of attorney not as support but as relinquishing power to me.

Looking at the empty sky as I sat next to my father in the Alzheimer's unit dining room, I remembered how much fear he'd had signing those medical powers of attorney. I guessed that the fear must be that much worse now, when he couldn't even understand what the paper meant. It struck me for the first time that he may not have understood exactly what the medical powers of attorney had meant, either. I felt ashamed for having bullied him into signing them. Nothing seemed to feel right anymore.

I put my hand on his and slowly repeated the daily litany. Did he understand any of it? Perhaps the sound of my voice, calm and reasonable, would make him feel more at home. "We think you had a stroke. Linda and I came back to Pennsylvania and brought you and Mom out to live near us in Idaho. Mom lives across the street, I live ten blocks away, and Linda is right outside town. We are moving your bank account out here so Mom can get at the money. Now, won't you sign it for me?"

At this last question, Dad peeked up sideways at me and took the pen. "Okay," he said, unexpectedly relaxed, his old handsome self.

"Right here on this line," I said, hopefully fixing my finger just above the spot.

And he signed . . . my name, Nancy C. Gerth. "There you go," he said proudly and set down the pen. He'd signed it "for me" all right.

I keep that form to remind me of the small victories of communication that can be achieved by those who are altered. Dad had made a joke, and in that moment, as his old self showed its face, he was pleased to have teased me into laughter. He was also pleased, I might add, to have won this one.

—*Nancy C. Gerth*

The Same, Only Different

My mother was rarely at a loss for words. If the right words didn't come to her, she would say something entirely inappropriate and take shocked silence at its face value, not seeming to understand that she'd offended her listeners. My siblings and I still talk about a toast she gave when my sister got engaged shortly after I had separated from my husband of eleven years. We gathered for a big family dinner and held our breaths when my mother rose, champagne glass in hand.

"I'd like to toast the beginning of one marriage and the end of another," she said.

The possibility that she might lose some of this verbal facility was not something I dreaded. Still, she was ridiculously young, only seventy-three, when she said to me during one of my visits, "Do you find me much changed?" She was shelling peas as we sat on the back porch, because she always did something else while talking. But I noticed that now she didn't shell and speak at the same time. Her glasses glinted as she turned her eyes to connect with mine.

"Changed? How? No," I said too quickly.

"I feel I've changed," she persisted. "Doesn't anything seem different to you? Do I seem a little slower to find the right words?"

"Well, sometimes," I acknowledged. "And you seem a little less steady on your feet."

I stopped and looked at her. She had turned her head away again and was staring at the bowl of peas. I still think of her as having dark hair and skin with a hint of olive, and I feel a fresh shock at the start of each visit to see how bleached out her coloring has become. Now, I could see her scalp, pale pink beneath thinning, white hair. I glanced away quickly, feeling queasy, as though I'd just seen the glistening gray-pink folds of her brain.

When I was a teen, I decided that aging must be an intensification of a personality's dominant trait—not so much a mellowing as a reducing that thickens the sauce and concentrates the flavor. My grandmother, for example, was a depressed and repressive woman in her prime, and as she aged, she became even darker. Her sister, lively and curious in her youth, became even more so in her later years. I had always expected my mother to carry on this tradition, and I dreaded what she might say. But something mysterious started happening. She struggled to find words, but all that came out were pauses filled with a crackling tension. She couldn't always follow the action in movies, because she'd forget which character was which. And when she asked me to take a look at the timeline she'd created as a starting point for her memoirs, I could not bring myself to speak. I simply changed dates in red ink. Grandmother didn't die in 1977, she died in 1980. I married in 1988, not 1992. Mom's first grandson was born in 1996, not 1990.

"At least," I said with black humor to my siblings, "there should be fewer tactless comments."

I spoke too soon. When I received her Christmas letter that year, I read that Claire had made a mistake in choosing her latest job and was now unemployed, David was doing nothing with his life, I was miserable and taken advantage of in my current relationship, and Joey, age nine, was entering kindergarten.

In the letter, she wrote much as she had always done, apart from occasional factual errors. The difference was more obvious when she tried to speak. The pauses were long, but they were only part of a larger change—my mother was no longer listening. Maybe it was her hearing problems, or maybe it was her preoccupation with her health. Maybe she chose not to listen because she didn't want to be drawn into conversations only to lose her verbal thread. I wanted to believe those explanations, because I didn't want to believe that my mother might not be the same person I had known for so long.

But she had changed. She suddenly quit the retirement support group she'd founded ten years earlier. This was a radical departure for someone who had always loved support groups, who had responded to every challenge in our lives—from writing a thesis to getting a divorce to raising children—with, "Maybe you should join a group!"

"They all talk about how grateful they are to have had each other's support and how meaningful their connection with the group is," she said, her sarcasm not completely hiding her envy.

Now, my mother avoids groups, passes up opportunities to comment on our plans, shows no interest in spending time with friends, and can't complete a sentence if she's doing anything else. The woman who learned to white-water kayak in her fifties and to windsurf in her sixties now loses her balance on escalators or while trying to hang a curtain. I hold her arm to help her into and out of the canoe, but she trembles with the effort and I do all the paddling.

She writes fragments of memoirs, because writing is easier than speaking, and then she shows them to me, because I encourage her. She keeps coming back to the same few stories, about the events that took place around the time of my birth. The passing of so many years has ground away many of the details, leaving only a bedrock of sadness—and blame. As I've always suspected, she saw my birth as the point at which my father turned away from us. He began coming home later and stopped playing with my older brothers. She decided it was because of me; he didn't care for girls. Between the lines of her stories I read that familiar unspoken accusation, the blame that has undermined every fresh beginning my mother and I have tried to make.

My mother hasn't written about my sister, Claire, but theirs would be a love story.

Claire can't bear to see what's happening. "She's not the same," she sobbed to me on the telephone one night. "Mom's already gone, and someone different is in her place."

My wary distance from my mother and my own motherhood give me a different perspective. I told Claire how much I'd loved to hold my babies and feel their soft, heavy bodies against me, their heads resting on my chest as they slept. I explained how they had changed every day, a little at a time, and now they prefer to spend time with friends and go off to camp without me, and sometimes they turn away from a good-night kiss.

"Everyone changes," I told her. "My sweet babies, stormy toddlers, and young children are gone. I see them only in flashbacks. The children here with me now have traits in common with my babies, but they're not the same. I'm always having to get to know and love them for who they are today. Maybe it would help if you could think of Mother that way."

"But Mom's not getting more capable every day," Claire pointed out. "It's not like babies at all. I want my old mom back."

"She's changed," I said. "And she'll keep changing. All we can do is get to know her, and love her, for who she is now."

So that's what we all try to do these days. It's not always easy to know and to love the person my mother is now. But then, it wasn't always easy to know and to love her as she was, either.

—Anne-Christine Strugnell

Respite from the Storm

Alzheimer's disease is slowly taking away my husband. There are still times when he returns and I remember what a magical love story Fred and I have lived for more than twenty years, though.

It's Writer's Club night. We meet for dinner at the Chowder Bowl and then move on to the library for our program. Fred, who volunteers at the Oregon Coast Aquarium, will join us at the restaurant after his shift.

The rain has finally stopped its attack. After pounding, pouring, flooding, and gusting for days, the air is still and a patch of palest blue peeks out of the white-gray clouds. As I turn onto the Coast Highway, I see the bottom of the sun hanging from a cloud like a yellow-gold Easter egg. As I drive, I keep looking west. Now there's the whole sun, stenciled with black Chinese characters.

Parking at the Nye Beach turnaround, I hurry to where I can see the horizon. Now the top of the Easter egg pokes up where the sea meets the sky. I have three minutes before I'm late to dinner, but I must watch as the sun slowly shrinks to a hyphen, then disappears. Tonight, instead of thinking, *Oh, it's gone, and now we will be immersed in darkness for the next fifteen hours,* I think about how the sun has gone to shine for someone else.

What does this have to do with Fred? Light. Hope. A respite from the storm. We have had some dark days lately—days when the man I loved was gone, replaced by a ghost who got lost in the middle of the night and stared at his cereal in the morning as if he didn't know what it was. But now, as I stand in that parking lot and inhale the sweet ocean air, I stretch and feel strong and alive from boots to fingertips. We will be all right.

At the Chowder Bowl, two newcomers are waiting. In a minute, my friend Carol arrives. Then our speaker, Cynthia, joins us, shaking hands all around. "I love this place," she says. "Did you see that sunset?"

Because it's winter and the tourists are gone, we have the restaurant to ourselves. We claim the big table in the corner.

As we talk, I keep looking out the window for Fred, relieved when I see our blue Mazda pickup glide by on its way to the parking lot. Midday, his stomach bothered him. He has been having some accidents lately, and I thought I might be called to the aquarium to bring clean pants. Then, despite the note I gave him, I worried he might forget about the meeting and sit at the house wondering where I was.

But here he is, all jingling aquarium badges. And he's handsome in his royal blue sweatshirt. As far as anyone can tell, I'm the woman with the greatest husband.

Carol knows of his illness but says nothing, just gives him a big hug. Cynthia may remember hearing about it, but the others have no idea and there's no need to mention it.

The waitress swings by. "Cannonball?" That's clam chowder in a big bread bowl with a shrimp salad on the side, Fred's usual. Menus confuse him, so he always orders the same thing.

"Yes. And coffee."

"Dressing?"

"Honey mustard." Usually, he says "um" and looks at me to finish the order, but tonight he remembers.

We eat and talk, our conversation dominated by the strangers, Suzy and Ron, mostly Suzy, who has taken too many writing workshops and goes on and on about them. Carol counters with stories about her workshops. Cynthia smiles indulgently. I watch my husband. Fred, who is not a writer, quietly listens and enjoys his chowder.

Eventually, the subject changes. It turns out that most of us are from California, and we discover that Fred and Suzy attended the same junior high and high schools in Burbank. Suzy was one year behind Fred. She names lots of names. Do you know . . . ? And he actually does know some of them. He's excited, speaking clearly. Alzheimer's destroys short-term memory, but his long-term memory is fine.

When the checks come, Fred silently slides ours over to me, and I figure out the tip, but he takes the money to the cash register.

By the time the rest of us get to the library, Fred and Carol are already there. Fred comes into the meeting room bearing paperbacks from the freebie shelf, hands them to me, and gets busy setting up the blue plastic chairs. He's a handy part of the team, my muscles.

I'm running the meeting, so I sit up front. Fred and Carol giggle in the back. The room fills to the point where I start wondering whether we'll run out of chairs, but we have just enough. After I do the intros, Cynthia jumps up and starts talking. Her style is fast and funny. In a minute, she has us on the ladder of humanity, from animalistic to Godlike, warning that, if the characters don't move on that ladder, nobody's going to be interested in the story. She describes cycles of creativity and tells secrets about selling scripts in Hollywood.

Cynthia has worked with famous producers, directors, and actors. She has been nominated for an Emmy. Yet, she's nobody's idea of a Hollywood shaker—not young, skinny, or stylish. She has a slew of grown children she raised alone, and she recently lost her mother to Alzheimer's. Through it all, she has lived the dream, and everyone in the room wants to do the same.

Now and then, I glance back and see Fred listening, smiling, laughing. God, he's mine. I am so lucky.

When the writer's meeting is over, Fred and the Depoe Bay postmaster stow the furniture back in the closet while the crowd trickles away. Nearly alone, I grab my husband for a long, sweet hug and kiss. I don't care if anyone sees us.

"I love you. I'm so glad you came," I tell him, and I mean it.

"It was fun," he says, and he means it.

He shouldn't be driving at night, but it isn't far and we take the chance. I follow him, grateful it's not raining.

As I watch Fred drive smoothly south on Highway 101, I think about how well he's doing. His official diagnosis was two years ago Saturday. Symptoms appeared three years before that. Yet, he is still driving, still volunteering at the aquarium, still able to show up and make my friends think I nabbed the best husband around. Tonight I have a partner, and it feels good.

Whatever happens in the future, I lucked out. We have had the kind of love most people never find. We have traveled the world together. Fred has supported me well, and he has always been my biggest fan. I am blessed, even if the ghost returns before the sun comes up, even if the next storm threatens to tear the roof off the house.

—*Sue Fagalde Lick*

In the Valley of Denial

A quick look down the street to make sure the coast was clear, a short sprint to the curb to retrieve my paper, and a mad dash back to the house—that was my game plan. I was loath to be seen in my shabby old robe and slipper-socks. If only the paperboy had a better throwing arm.

It was unusual for me to take a sick day, but, boy, did I need one today. Hot flashes and night sweats had kept me awake for hours, and I was dead tired. Just the thought of getting dressed and fighting traffic was enough to make me sick.

"Gooooood mooooooorning!" The voice sang out over the fence that separated our properties.

Damn! Where did she come from? I live next door to the town watch. Think my life is easy? Sheila has a heart of gold, but she's nosy as hell with a mouth as big as Texas. What could I do? I invited her in for coffee.

She got right to the point. "You need to do something about your mother."

"What're you talking about?"

"She's losing it."

After years of being neighbors, she still gets under my skin.

"I saw her in Strawbridge's Monday. I went over to say hello, and she just stared at me. I swear she didn't even—"

I pushed down on the coffee grinder; it made a satisfyingly loud racket.

"—know who I was."

She didn't miss a beat. "I said, 'Ruth, remember me, Sheila? I live next door to Gail.'"

Why didn't I go into work today?

"She looked frightened. I asked her if Eddie was with her, and she said he was outside but she couldn't find the door."

"My brother takes good care of her since my father died."

"He can't see the forest for the trees. He's too close to her. But I gave him a piece of my mind when I found him sitting in his car. Told him he shouldn't let her go into the store alone. He wasn't too happy with me."

Why didn't Eddie tell me about this?

"I'll definitely talk to him."

Truth be told my brother and I didn't talk much. The only time I saw him was when he brought Mom for a visit or to holiday dinner.

We were never close. I was five when he was born. My mother fussed over him like he was a porcelain doll. At six he suffered complications after a tonsillectomy and spent several months in the hospital. My parents spent most of their time at his bedside. I spent most of my time with neighbors. When he came home, I felt excluded from all the attention surrounding him.

My parents became more protective, and I turned rebellious. Typical mother–daughter conflicts turned into full-fledged war. When Dad was home, he pulled combat duty and became the mediator. If he sided with me, Mom got mad and didn't speak to him for days. If he took her side, I wouldn't speak to either of them.

My teenage years were spent wishing Mom was someone else's mother. She must have felt the same. All through high school she encouraged me to get married. I was only too happy to comply.

My brother never left the nest. When Dad died, he lost his best friend. If anything happened to our mother, he'd be alone.

She had been forgetful lately. She'd ask the same question repeatedly until I was ready to scream.

And sometimes she couldn't find the right word to express herself, but it didn't seem too out-of-line for an eighty-year-old. Hopefully, she'd just had a senior moment in the department store.

But the following week I received a disturbing phone call.

"Where are you?"

"I'm at work, Mom; you called my office."

"I can't do it."

"Do what?"

"The thing you put food in doesn't turn. He'll get mad."

"I'll call Eddie at work. He won't be mad." I hope.

Mom was right about one thing: Eddie was mad. He claimed she was being ornery and wouldn't follow simple directions. When I asked about the department store incident, the flood gates opened: "Sheila should mind her own business." "She exaggerates." "Mother was tired." "I get lost in stores too." Yada, yada, yada.

As I listened to his diatribe, it occurred to me that he may have been covering up her lapses for a long time.

At least Eddie agreed that Mom should see a specialist.

The neurosurgeon was highly recommended. His waiting room was packed. We sat in a row, Eddie and I flanking Mom like we were the parents. I wasn't sure she knew where she was.

The physical was brief. Her primary-care doctor had already done blood work, an EEG, and an MRI. Today, there would be a psychological exam consisting of a series of questions:

"What is today's date?"

"Repeat after me: ball, tree, pen."

"Spell 'world' backward."

"What building are we in?"

Mom answered some of the questions but was silent for others. Later in the exam, the doctor asked her to recall the three words. I could see her groping for them, but they were out of reach. I wanted to blurt them out for her, but I bit my tongue.

At last, it was over.

"I'm fairly certain she's in the middle stages of Alzheimer's disease."

The words were shocking. This had always been a possibility, but it hadn't been real until now.

"I'm prescribing donepezil. It's not a cure. Maybe it'll buy us some time."

He looked at me sympathetically, but I was angry. He had no right to use the word "us." We weren't talking about his mother.

"There may be a breakthrough. . . ."

I felt thankful that my mother didn't seem to realize she had just been handed a death sentence.

Eddie shook his head. "This is bullshit! A diagnosis by asking a few questions? Hell, I couldn't even answer half of them."

I wondered what it would take to convince him, but I didn't try. He needed time to digest the news. We should have been making plans, but that could wait. I wasn't anxious to think about the future either.

The phone calls became more frequent. Mom can't work the appliances. She heard a cat in the basement. Eddie threatened to put her in a nursing home. . . .

I got into the habit of stopping by their house after work. Some days, she was fine; other days, not so fine.

One day I let myself in and found the television playing to an empty living room. I called out; no one answered. Worried, I ran upstairs to check the bedrooms. Mom was sitting on the bed. Her clothes were wrinkled, and she looked like she needed a bath. She didn't make any sense.

"You know, uh, dogs can't see inside her house bark."

I did hear barking. A light bulb went off. I flew down the steps. Sure enough, the barking came from the TV. I didn't know whether to laugh or cry. Instead, I turned off the TV and went back upstairs to help my mother bathe.

Her speech was word salad. Simple tasks were beyond her. Soon, she'd require constant supervision. It was past time to do something; still, I put it off.

Another week went by. Mom left the house on her own with no purse or keys. Disoriented, she walked a few blocks and fell. Fortunately, a neighbor rescued her, and she only suffered a bruised knee.

I wanted to stick my head in the sand like my brother. I wanted to scream at him: "She lives with you! Take better care of her!" I wanted to cry, "Why me?"

It was all so overwhelming. I'd hoped to retire in the near future and enjoy the rest of my life. Suddenly, my golden years were looking tarnished. I knew that other baby boomers with aging parents were going through similar circumstances, but each situation is unique, and mine was complicated by a brother in denial. Maybe I wasn't facing reality either. It was easier to go along with Eddie's course of action—or inaction—than to make some tough decisions. My deeply buried resentment was keeping me from doing what needed to be done. She was not my brother's sole responsibility because he lived with her; she was my mother, too.

Mom and I had never spoken of the past. Now, it was too late. Pretty soon she wouldn't even know who I was. I needed to clear my head of old history and past hurts, and I'd have to do it myself.

I let go of my idealized vision of "motherhood" and concentrated on accepting Mom as the woman she was—one who made mistakes, a lot like me. I had always faulted her for putting her parents in a nursing home. It was time to relinquish blame. She'd done the best she could. I came to realize she was a mother who cared deeply but didn't know how to show it. There would be no happy ending for us, but at least I could face her needs with love instead of resentment.

My husband and I knew what we wanted to do, but we needed to get my brother on board.

We dropped the bomb on Eddie. "We want to move her into our house. The in-law suite is perfect, everything on one floor. I know someone who can watch her during the day."

"You're taking my mother away."

"No. Alzheimer's is taking her away. We need to keep her safe and comfortable as long as we can."

"I want to help out."

"I'll give you a key to our house. We can do this together. It'll be okay."

He smiled at me.

I think it really will be okay.

—*Gail Pruszkowski*

The Other Woman

The first thing I notice about the rest home's dining room is that Mom is not at her regular table. She usually sits next to her wheelchair-bound friend, Miss Margaret. Then she can push Miss Margaret's water glass closer so she can reach it, ask questions Miss Margaret nods and grunts to, and wipe off her clothes when the peas or applesauce in Miss Margaret's spoon don't quite reach her mouth. But this morning Mom is at the aides' table with her arms crossed and her lips pressed together.

"Oh, there you are." She looks me up and down. By the clarity and strength in her voice, I know she is agitated.

I pat her hands and hug her shoulders, trying to give her as much body contact as possible. This was something Aunt Clara suggested on the phone last night. "People with Alzheimer's feel cut off from the world," she said. "Lots of touching and hugging helps calm them down." I didn't like having my mom referred to as one of "them," but I knew Aunt Clara was trying to help.

The changes in my mother have been hard to accept. A kind and sensitive woman, she used to spend her days writing articles for the local newspaper, visiting friends, walking along the sound, or reading to a class of elementary school kids. Recently, she has gone from forgetting what time and day it is to forgetting how to clothe and bathe herself. The first time I saw her come out of her room with nothing on but her jeans and bra, I thought maybe she'd forgotten that my husband was in the house with me. But when she made her way through the living room and reached for the knob on the front door, saying, "I'm going to walk down to the lake," I knew something was very wrong. The lake she was referring to is Lake George, located in upstate New York. It is beside her parents' old summer cottage, a thousand miles away from where she now lives in North Carolina. I kept Mom from leaving the house and directed her back to the bedroom, where I helped her into a sweatshirt. But over the next couple of weeks her mood deteriorated until she was constantly anxious and agitated, the way she appears now.

"They all know." She cocks her head at the tables of people around her.

"Who? What do they know?" I don't really want her to answer, but she has caught me off guard.

"They know what your father's been doing. How he's been going out on me."

"What do you mean? Daddy has been back at the house, snoring on his bed or watching TV in his lounge chair during our entire visit."

As far as I can tell, my dad leaves the house only to have lunch at the senior center or an early dinner at the hospital cafeteria before visiting Mom. He seems worn out from months of doing all the grocery shopping and preparing meals, not to mention being the target of Mom's emotional outbursts when he reminds her it is impossible to go see her mother because she's been dead for twenty years. Even though he is in the last stages of prostate cancer, he promised her he'd take care of her as long as he was alive. The rest of my family and I were able to convince him that Mom needed to be in a place where she could receive more care only after her family doctor recommended she be hospitalized for neurological testing, and the neurologist insisted that it wasn't safe for her to return home.

"You know, that woman. Margo, the sexy one. I'd like to give her something to think about, like a punch in the mouth."

The anger, the reference to sex, this is not Mom speaking. She's never raised her hand to anyone in her life. Nor have I ever heard her accuse Daddy of being unfaithful. I clasp her hand and try to think of something to say that will change the subject as I glance around the room for anyone who might fit the bill of sexy. About thirty women, all over the age of eighty, are sprinkled about the cafeteria finishing their breakfasts.

Could she be referring to one of the aides? Three of them sit around the table, oblivious to my mother's words. They are dressed in boxy, pale green and white outfits, hunched over their food.

"Let's go back to your room. I think Daddy may be waiting to visit."

"He is?" Her voice is unsteady, and her eyes flick up at me for a half second. "How do you know?"

"Trust me," I say. This morning, on our way out of town, I drove my father over to the rest home, and my husband followed behind in our Blazer. While Daddy came inside with me, Joel chose to stay in the truck and read the paper.

"He's probably waiting there to tell me what to do," Mom says now. "Or maybe he's looking for my money."

The switch is so sudden, I'm almost thrown. Rubbing her forearm, I guide her down the hall. Her steps are small, and her upper body leans forward. I adjust my hold on her arm to keep her from toppling over. For a moment, I remember how it used to be, how she was the one who did the supporting, And I was the stiff child she'd hold in her arms. She'd stroke my hair until I leaned my head against her shoulder and let the tears flow.

"Mom, I know Daddy loves you."

"Yeah, sure he does. Why's he going around with that woman?"

"I promise you . . ." We pause in the hall, and I squeeze her hand and kiss her cheek, where the skin is pale and papery. "He's not doing that. He loves you."

We walk on and reach her room. Daddy is lying on her couch watching TV.

Her face crumples. "Yeah—so much that he leaves me here and tries to steal my money."

Daddy is sitting up now, nervously glancing toward us. "Hey, Bet. How are you?"

I know he hopes the sight of him will cheer her up. Last night he told me she had held onto his arms and begged him not to leave.

Mom stalks by him into her bedroom. Motioning to Daddy, I follow her and guide us to a seat on the bed. Daddy sits in a chair near her. She has said she wants us to talk honestly and openly.

"Daddy, Mom is worried. She thinks you're taking her money." I stroke her arm and glance back and forth between them. Mom is staring at Daddy as if he has the power to change everything. "Do you have any money on you? Maybe you could give Mom some of what you have."

Daddy squints. Mom's disease makes no sense to him. Instead of trying to make her feel better, my father usually tries to defend himself, which only upsets her further. I keep telling him to respond to her feelings. Today, I hope he'll follow my lead.

Finally, he reaches into his pocket and pulls out a money clip. "I have five—no, ten—dollars." He holds up two five-dollar bills. "Here, Bet, I'll give you one and keep one. Now, you've got just as much as I do."

I know he's trying. But despite her illness, Mom knows when my father is being condescending. Still, I hope the gesture will mean something. She looks down, pressing her lips together. Her chin is trembling.

"I'm just afraid you've left me here, and you're going off to be with those other women."

I knew money wasn't the issue. My father clumsily pats her arm. After talking with Aunt Clara last night, I tried to school him on the importance of touching and not getting upset when she sounds unreasonable. But I can see his tolerance is waning as he glances at his watch. It's past nine; we're going to miss the game. My husband and I had planned to stop by the gym to see my eight-year-old nephew play basketball on our way out of town. Daddy was counting on it. I'm not sure I can leave.

"You go on. I'll meet you there," I say to him. This is code for "you leave first, and I'll meet you in the car if I can get away."

My mother's intuition is right. There is something strange going on. But it's not what she thinks. The other woman my father is spending time with is me. I've spent more time with my father and spoken to him more on the phone in the last couple of months than I have in the last ten years. As Mom's mind began slipping, he became my main source of information, and I became one of his main sources of support.

But there aren't words to explain this to Mom without upsetting her. She knows she feels different, but she's insulted if I use the words Alzheimer's or dementia. The times I have gently explained her condition, she nods with a questioning look in her eyes. A few seconds later, she'll ask, "What did you say my problem was?"

I sit quietly for a moment, stroking Mom's hand, tracing the lines on her palm.

"I hate to say this, Mom, but Joel and I have to go home today."

She presses her lips tight again and wipes a tear from her lashes. "I just wish . . ." her voice fades off. "I wish I could go with you."

An aide peeks in the door. She smiles and waves when she sees me. I wave back.

"I hate this place," Mom says. "They're all smiles and laughs, but you know something else is going on."

I wonder if she has forgotten that I have to go or if my words even registered. It's so unlike my mother not to listen. All my life she was the one who listened to every story I brought home from school. She'd spend hours with her head laid back on the green cushion in the chair in the kitchen, absorbing every word about my teachers, my friends, my dreams—never judging, always interested. It's still a shock when she doesn't hear me now.

She looks straight ahead at the photograph of Lake George I had enlarged for her. I had hoped the familiar blue water surrounded by rolling mountains would be soothing. Now I wonder if she thinks I'm going there without her.

Over the next few minutes I try to say good-bye without upsetting her. I tell her I'll call when I get home and that my brother will be by to visit later.

My voice is unnaturally cheery in an effort to elevate her mood, the one last thing I think I can give her before I leave. She doesn't say her usual words, "I'll be okay. Have a good trip, and thanks for everything." She doesn't say, "It's been lovely to see you, dear."

I stand up slowly. The muscles in my hamstrings and calves tighten as I bend over to kiss her cheek. There's a smudge of toothpaste on her chin, and faint lines of lipstick run up the creases of her mouth. At the last moment she turns her head, pursing her lips. Mine brush hers in a gesture we've never shared. I wonder if she thinks I'm Daddy. Just in case, I put my arms around her shoulders and hold her extra close.

—Ann Campanella

This story was first published in the May 2004 issue of Today's Charlotte Woman *magazine.*

Lost and Found

My father is missing. It was my decision to put him in a home, and I chose this particular home for its reputation for working with people with Alzheimer's. Now, my father has gone missing. The caretaker at the home told me over the phone that they suspect he walked out the front door while a delivery was being made. They think he is out walking around the city somewhere. I thought my father would be safe there. I was the one who wanted him there the most. I pushed and pushed until I got my way. Now I don't know where he is.

When I walk into the nursing home, I realize that I have lost my father for the second time in my life. The first time was when I walked out of my parents' home at the age of sixteen. I wanted nothing to do with him. I felt I could keep walking forever and never look back. Now, I seem to do a great deal of looking back, and with his Alzheimer's, so does my father. As I sign myself in at the reception desk, I realize how foolish I was back then and feel my face burn with shame. Although it is painful to relive old memories, I am not sixteen anymore, even though my father sometimes thinks I am. Now, I see things differently.

Walking into my father's room, where I'll meet with the director to talk about what happened with my father over the last few hours, I think back to my conversation with Tina that finally convinced her to let me put Dad in the nursing home.

Tina is my father's wife of twenty-seven years. They met, fell in love, and got married between my first and second year of elementary school. He was still married to my mom for part of that time. When I was fifteen, my mom died, and I moved in with Dad and Tina. It was a new city, a new school, and a new family. I didn't handle it well. Looking back, I recognize other times where I may not have handled things well, including the time I talked to Tina about putting Dad in the home.

"Tina, you said yourself that he can go for days at a time not knowing who you are, that he thinks your dog, Major, is his long lost dog, Blackie, from when he was six."

"It isn't that bad; it's just now and then." Tina didn't want to admit Dad to a nursing home. Tina didn't want to admit there was a problem at all.

"You just told me that he calls you Ellen, my mother's name!" I said a bit too loudly.

"I can take care of him," she said, not looking at me.

As I sat at her kitchen table drinking her watery coffee, I found myself wondering if she had resented me for encroaching on her partnership with my dad after my mother died. I wondered if she resented me now for suggesting we put him in a home, ultimately forcing their separation.

"No, Tina, you can't take care of him," I said more gently. "That is part of the reason why this is so important. He is going to get worse; he is going to lose control of himself. You can't do it all alone. You still see him as Daniel, your husband."

"Of course, I see him as Daniel! Who is he, if not Daniel?"

"I'm sorry. I don't mean to say he is someone else; of course he's not."

"Of course he's not," she repeated. "He's my husband. He's my Daniel."

"But not in the way he was, not in any way you can rely on," I said.

She looked at me now, an expression of fear and grief shadowing her face. I paused—knowing how difficult this was for her to understand and accept. It was for me, too. I took a deep breath and then continued in a calm voice.

"This disease, Alzheimer's, has slowly taken him over. It will only get harder, both for Dad and for you. I'm sorry, Tina, but he isn't really your Daniel now, and he will become less so as time goes on."

My stepmother looked away in sudden recognition of the truth of my words. She silently sipped her coffee while I went on.

"He's all the Daniels he's ever been. He's Daniel, the young man who gets into fist fights with guys at the bar. He's Daniel, the six-year-old searching for his lost dog. He's Daniel, Ellen's husband, before he met you." This last part I say into my coffee cup, not trusting my emotions.

"He would not want to go into a home," Tina said pointedly.

"You're right, he wouldn't," I acknowledged. "But this isn't up to Dad. And it isn't up to you either. He gave me power of attorney."

"He gave that to you in case something happened to us both, not so you could override my decisions about what is best for him," she says without a trace of testiness. Tina really is a remarkable woman.

"That may be so, but this is what is best for him—and for you. It will only tear you down to keep on living moment to moment, not knowing which Daniel is sitting in front of you."

I had researched this. I had visited several nursing homes. "Tina," I said quietly but firmly, "you have to trust me. This is the right place for Dad."

She said nothing. Taking her silence as a sign that she was beginning to accept my plan, I pushed forward.

"We can admit him on the first of the month. They will have an apartment available then. It has a living room and an eat-in kitchen, and the bedroom is separate. I've seen it. It is lovely. He'll be happy there."

"He is happy here," she says, her resolve beginning to falter.

"Yes, but not for long. As he progresses, he'll need to be around what is familiar. If we wait much longer, it will be too late and he won't feel comfortable in any facility, because he won't be able to connect it to anything."

Once again, I was met with silence. I had to convince her, so I continued to press the matter.

"We have to take him there now, so that he can adjust and feel at home."

"He is at home here."

"Yes, for now, but when it becomes too much for you—and it will become too much for you—"

I stopped, realizing I was pushing too hard. I could tell by the way she was fussing with her coffee cup. She wasn't looking at me anymore, either.

"At some point, he'll have to be admitted to a
home. Doing it now is in his best interest."

I paused, determined to wait until she acknowledged what I'd said. I couldn't bully her into this; he
would not want that. Several minutes passed, and
finally she nodded.

As I stand alone in my father's living room at the nursing home, I am uncertain if I've made the right choice,
and I am left to wonder where he could have gone. I begin
to examine his possessions, searching for a clue.

"Mrs. Kuskovski?" the director walks into the
room, pulling me back from my memories. "It is good
to see you again. Thank you for coming so quickly."

"Do you have any idea where he may have gone?"
I ask.

"That is what we were hoping to ask you."

"I . . . I don't know," I manage to stammer, my eyes
stinging with tears. "He couldn't have gone far; he was
discovered missing only an hour ago, correct?"

She hands me a tissue and guides me to a chair.
"Yes, and we have the police looking for him."

"Have you called his wife, Tina?" I ask, thinking I'll bring Tina to my place tonight. There is no
way she'll get through the night alone not knowing
where he is and whether he's okay.

"Yes, of course, but there was no answer."

The director assures me that every available staff member and three squad cars are all looking for my father. I get up from my chair to resume searching for some clue as to where my father may have gone. With my back to the door, I hear it open. Assuming it is the director leaving the room, I am quite surprised when I hear a friendly bark of recognition from my father's four-year-old black lab, Major, who begins nuzzling and licking my hand. I turn around and see, to my relief, that my father is standing in the doorway. Tina is behind him.

When my father was six, his dog was hit and killed by a car, but his parents told him the dog must have run away. My dad had gone out searching for Blackie every evening for close to a year. My grandparents never got him another dog; aware that he'd never really gotten over the loss of Blackie, they were afraid to put him through that again should anything happen to a new dog. Of course, my dad had seen it differently, and though the other dogs he'd had as an adult all had more inspired names, they were all black labs in honor of Blackie.

Now, when my dad regresses to the six-year-old Daniel, he resumes his search for Blackie. This time, his search had taken him twenty miles away to the home he'd shared with Tina to retrieve Major, the black lab he'd gotten before Alzheimer's began to steal his short-term memory. Confusing Major for Blackie is a lapse he'd repeat often.

It was quite difficult for Tina to get my father and Major to settle down enough for the forty-five-minute car ride back to the nursing home. From the red rims of her eyes, I can tell it has taken its toll on her.

As we sit down with the director to talk things over, my father doesn't seem to notice. He is a six-year-old boy, overcome with joy at having found his beloved Blackie. Tina is forthcoming about her concerns for taking care of Dad on her own. I am relieved to hear this, and we agree to keep him at the home. But, we are all still concerned about his having gotten so far on his own and are unsure how to proceed.

In the end, the director, Tina, and I agree to have my dad continue living at the home, provided Major is able to stay with him.

My father continues to have lucid days and days when he is lost to us on many levels, but he no longer goes missing. Tina and I have grown considerably closer and are better able to communicate than we were before. The two of us make decisions about Dad's care in partnership now. We don't always agree on everything, but as far as putting my dad in the home when we did, that is one decision we are both glad to have made. As for Major, he brings smiles to more than one patient at the home, regardless of what name they may call him.

—*Jennifer Kuskovski*

I Am My Mother's Daughter, After All

My mother was named Miss Popularity of Steelton, Pennsylvania, in 1931. The prize photo of her—in a lush, white fur jacket, standing on a tiger skin rug (head and all!), half hidden behind a gigantic bouquet of roses—hangs in my bedroom.

Seventeen at the time of her "popularity," Juliana Gabner was the oldest girl among seven surviving siblings. She "worked" in the neighborhood general store when she was ten years old and was paid with bags of penny candy, which her mother made her share with her sisters and brothers. She quit school in the seventh grade because her younger sister was promoted a year and she didn't want to be in the same class with her. Mom lied about her age and got a paying job when she was just thirteen. At twenty-one, she met my father, fell in love, and married him after only two months. Throughout her life, my mother was lovely, gregarious, charming, and generous. She was always entertaining—holiday dinners, costume parties, sing-alongs, summer barbecues, and fireworks on the Fourth of July.

I was not like my mother. We rarely saw eye to eye on anything. She wanted me to be popular and date boys; I chose to go to an all girls' high school. She wanted me to get a job and earn money; I went to college. She wanted me to live at home until I married; I went to Africa. (It was the sixties, and President Kennedy had just started the Peace Corps; I thought I'd go save the world from poverty.) I was more like my dad, quiet and never wanting to be in the spotlight. When he died in 1973, I was devastated. My mother bounced back much faster than I did.

It wasn't until many years after I left home, when I took a Myers-Briggs Personality Inventory, that I discovered my mother and I were polar opposites: she, an extroverted social butterfly who needed lots of friends around all the time; I, an introvert who would rather spend a whole day in bed with a book than get dressed and go out even to the grocery store. I understood then that we couldn't help being so different. She surely had as much trouble accepting me as her daughter as I did accepting her as my mother. It was sometime after my fiftieth birthday that we began to tolerate one another.

My mother had never been sick in all her eighty years. The only time she'd seen a doctor was when she had to take my sister or me to one, and the only time she'd been hospitalized was to give birth to us. But the summer I turned fifty, during a two-week visit to her new home on the East Coast, I arrived just in time to rush her to the emergency room. She had pneumonia.

A nurse came into the little cubicle to take her health history. "Do you wear glasses?" No. "Hearing aid?" No. "False teeth?" No. "Heart trouble, diabetes, ever had a stroke?" No. No. No. The no's went down the entire list of possible conditions and diseases that an eighty-year-old woman might have. "And how often do you have your period?" the nurse asked. My mother laughed along with my sister and me. "Well, everything else is still working," the nurse said, "so I thought that must be, too."

My mother quickly recovered from the pneumonia and resumed her normal life . . . or so we thought.

My sister and I didn't notice anything different about her for a year or so. Then, every time I visited, she was more forgetful, more confused, and less "herself," except when she was with her great-grandson. With Aaron, she played like a child herself, chasing him around the dining room table; singing nurs-

ery rhymes; making faces with raisins on his pea-
nut butter sandwiches; dressing up in funny clothes;
and holding, hugging, kissing, and loving him every
minute.

By the time Aaron's little sister was born three
years later, she could hold the baby only if she were
sitting down with one of us right next to her to help.
She had "forgotten" how to hold the bottle, how to
change a diaper, how to sing lullabies to a baby. She
no longer cooked, not even her famous baked pork
chops that everyone praised. She got dressed, bathed,
and washed her hair only if one of us helped her.
(Although she still wanted us to apply the auburn
hair coloring she had started using years before!)
She'd stopped writing letters to her friends, and even
when I wrote out the addresses, she could barely sign
her name to Christmas cards. It wasn't Alzheimer's,
the doctor said, just "aging," just "dementia."

My mother still lived alone in her condo. She
never turned on the gas stove or tried to flush her
underwear down the toilet. But if I was cooking
something and left the kitchen for a minute, she
would turn off the stove. And she started putting
toilet paper in a wastebasket so as not to plug the
toilet. Then the evening anxiety began, "sundown-
ers" as the medical community calls it. She would
phone my sister or my sister's daughter or son or even

me halfway across the county. "I need help," she'd whimper. "I can't breathe. Come here and help me," she'd plead. "I need you."

One of them would rush over and find her taking a walk outside or watching television or sleeping—nothing wrong. She called twenty, thirty times a day. After a while, they stopped answering their phones. My sister began to go to our mother's house every night after work and have supper with her and sleep there. In the mornings, Mom would be okay, but by late afternoon, it all started again.

One day my mother fell while walking outside. A neighbor heard her cries and called an ambulance and then my sister. She wasn't badly hurt, but we knew we had to do something now. Neither my sister nor I could quit our jobs or stop helping our children and grandchildren, so we found an assisted-living home a few blocks away from the condo she'd lived in since my father's death. We hoped she'd adjust and be glad to have people around her again. The other residents and staff were caring and cheerful and tried to make her feel at home. But she wasn't home, and she knew it, and she wasn't happy about it.

Now, all she wants is to go back home. When I visit her the first thing she says is, "Am I going home with you?" Once there I can't leave, because she cries, gets angry, and yells at me, "Then don't ever come back." So I sit by her bed, my arm stretched over her shoulders and my feet up by hers, and tell her I'm in the bed with her and staying all night. After she falls asleep, I tiptoe out and leave, knowing I must return the next morning before she wakes up.

Although I stay for two weeks at a time, each day when I arrive is the first time for her. She is surprised and delighted to see me, introduces me to everyone as her "baby" (I'm the younger child), asks me the same questions she asked a hundred times the day before and the day before that and the day before that.

When I'm with my mother, I bathe her. It took a while for me to get up the nerve to wash all of her body, but she doesn't mind my touching her. She won't use the bathtub or shower, so I gently wash and rinse her, then quickly dry her to avoid hearing, "Oh, it's so cold. Cover me up." I massage lotion into her paper-thin skin, oh so gently, so as not to bruise her. She is only skin and bones now, and even a light touch can hurt. I massage her gnarled feet, gently separating each toe. I dress her in the new clothes my sister is always buying for her, as if she were going to live forever. Mom still insists on wearing her bra, and I struggle to keep her shrunken breasts in while I close the hooks. Her bras are ancient, just threads held together by loose elastic. I bought her new ones, but she won't wear them. "Too tight," she says. I comb her now white hair, still with its little wave on the side, and then we walk.

My mother, who never just "went for a walk" in her life, now walks incessantly. When she was still in her own home, we walked outside, always the same route around the condo parking lot. Every time she'd say, "Why do those dandelions grow only on my front yard?" Then she'd count them, again pointing out that there were none on the neighbor's yard. And every time I'd promise to dig them out for her.

Now, in her assisted-living home, she walks only inside, down the hallway, through the living room and TV room, back to the dining room and kitchen. I walk with her, my arm around her back, taking infinitesimally small steps and stopping after each one. It can take us an hour to make the trek once through the home. We say the same things to each other over and over. She has begun to ask me why: "Why does my back hurt like this?" "Why am I so tired?" "Why am I here in this place?" "Why do you have to leave?" "Why can't you stay with me?" *Like a three-year-old*, I think, *always asking "why" until you get tired of it and say "because."*

Yes, I realize, *she is like a three-year-old, and I am her mother now.* This thought stuns me. I am doing for her all the things she did for me when I was young. I remember how she bathed me every evening before my father came home from work. I stood on the toilet seat cover while she scrubbed the day's play dirt from my elbows and knees as I whined, "It's too cold." She dressed me in pink pinafores, combed my hair and tried, hopelessly, to keep a satin bow in it. We walked to the corner to meet my father's bus and walked back home together. She cooked my food, washed my clothes, cleaned the house, took me to the toilet until I could do it myself—all those things that I now do for her.

For the first time, I realize how much my mother loved me and how much alike we really are. Now when I bathe her, I feel her hands washing me. When I dress her, I feel the blouse slip over my head. When we walk together, I am on the sidewalk in front of my childhood home, picking our dandelions. When I rub her aching back, I am in her arms again, feeling her firm, warm hands on my back.

Myers-Briggs was wrong. In our love for one another, my mother and I are more alike.

—*Kathleen M. Moore*

I Can Chase Lions

When my car's radiator hose burst at the summit of Colorado's Wolf Creek Pass in a foggy blizzard, I should have known what the rest of that trip would be like. But like the postman, I'd go through rain, snow, sleet, and even hail to keep my promise to fly my parents to their Pennsylvania home for a month-long visit. *How different will Dad be since I had seen him ten months ago?* I wondered.

Three years earlier, Dad had been diagnosed with Alzheimer's disease, though the first signs had appeared at least ten years before that. The symptoms manifested in a slow progression. "Gee, isn't Dad's memory getting bad?" my four sisters and I would ask each other. The memory loss grew to be a source of frustration. Then he forgot our names. He lost things and thought someone had stolen them.

He repeated the same questions. He began to wander in the woods nearby and imagine that he had talked to strangers.

Eventually, the stress grew too great for Mom, so my husband, two children, and I moved from Colorado to Pennsylvania, where we rented a trailer just up the road from my parents' country home. Besides Dad having Alzheimer's, both of my parents were in poor health. Dad had had a triple bypass, a back operation, and colon cancer. Mom had a weak heart, diabetes, and a nervous condition. Dad had to quit driving and hunting. He went from knowing me sometimes to often thinking that I, his fourth daughter, was his brother, who had died in World War II.

We'd been in Pennsylvania for a few years when my sister Linda invited our parents to live with her family in Sterling, Nebraska. Another sister, Judy, lived in nearby Lincoln and would be of help to Mom and Dad as well. That freed my family to return to Colorado.

Now, I was on my way to Nebraska with my kids, and then on to Pennsylvania with my parents. When we finally arrived at Linda's house, Dad hugged us as we told him who we were. Seeing how much his condition had degenerated disheartened me. He paced more, wandering from room to room, and had more difficulty with his balance. My brother-in-law redirected Dad by asking him to visit with us. Mike had volunteered to stay with Dad for a few hours while Mom and the others attended my nieces' homeschool program. Dad didn't ask where his wife, Ginny, was, as he used to.

"We came a long way to see you, Dad," I explained. "Ginny and I will take you to Pennsylvania."

"I've heard of that place," he said of the state he had lived in for more than seventy years.

At times he stared vacantly, playing with his belt, but then he'd look up and smile at my children. He pointed to our suitcases. "Aren't they nice?" he asked. It was his way of making conversation. The present moment and what was in front of him were his only world. I felt as if Dad had already died. I could hardly remember what he was like before the disease.

Soon the rest of the family returned from the school program, and we packed my parents' suit-cases for the next day. My children would stay in Sterling while I took my parents to Pennsylvania. A multitude of things could go wrong on the long and complicated trip. *Is taking this trip pure insanity?* I wondered.

It seemed that way when Dad was admitted into the hospital the next morning with stomach cramps. In all the excitement, he hadn't been eating right, which clog his bowels. During the next week, he proved to be an escape artist: undoing his restraints, pulling out the intravenous lines, and removing the tube in his throat many times during the night. Mom and I would fall asleep in the chairs by Dad's bed. Worry about his health dominated her conversation.

Magnifying the Twilight-Zone feeling, the nurses insisted we stay in the bathroom during a tornado warning. Dad's chair fit in the shower and Mom's by the light switch; the toilet sufficed as my seat. With knees touching, we passed the forty-five minutes counting money, Dad counting all bills as ones. He didn't seem to notice anything unusual about the accommodations.

When our second departure date arrived, we made up our mind to go at the last minute. We rushed to the Lincoln airport and boarded the small plane just in time. At the Minneapolis layover, we smuggled Dad into the women's restroom, where we could help him, and then in the waiting area he ate his submarine sandwich one layer at a time.

My sister Kathy picked us up in Cleveland and drove us to her home in Youngstown. The next morning, on the way to Pennsylvania, we stopped at a little restaurant for lunch. Kathy and I watched as Dad carefully spread his applesauce on his grilled-cheese sandwich. We glanced at each other, mouths twitching, anticipating his first bite. He took off the top with the applesauce and ate the bottom part. Kathy's and my sides shook as we snorted and snuffled, trying to maintain composure.

When we pulled up to my parents' home, Dad stared blankly at the house. The grass needed mowing, which looked strange because Dad had always kept the grass cut to the nubbins. I wondered if he'd want to mow again. He looked at his mower as if he were seeing it for the first time and said, "That's nice. I think I'll use it someday."

The next day I looked out the window and spied Dad trying to mow the lawn with the wheelbarrow.

"Ginny! What's wrong with this thing?" he asked.

Mom tried to tell him. Then, in despair, she ran into the house. I watched as he tried to cut the grass. He stopped, circling the wheelbarrow, muttering and frowning. He knew something was wrong. Finally, he gave up and put it away. I wasn't sure how he'd do with a real lawnmower, so I didn't show him how to use it. The next day he tried to rake the yard with a mop. I gave him the rake. He wouldn't hurt himself with that.

From then on Dad puttered in the yard. One day I watched as he jumped across the ditch. He'd forgotten where the bridge was. He leaped surprisingly well.

"You're in good shape for the shape you're in," I told him.

I showed him the bridge. Surprisingly, he remembered it after that. While Dad worked, I caught a glimpse of the way he used to be. He had always been active—hunting, fishing, and working.

His diet presented another concern, but sometimes our best efforts were for nothing. Since Dad now had to avoid excess roughage, he was hungry all the time. To compound the problem, he would forget that he had already eaten. One evening he ate a huge sticky bun. Then half an hour later he wanted another one. Concerned about all the sugar, Mom handed him half. He insisted on the whole one. He looked like a little kid, smiling mischievously as he carted off his prize. One time I picked out all the forbidden fresh tomatoes from his salad and returned them to the serving bowl. After eating his salad, he proceeded to eat the tomatoes out of the remaining salad.

Sometimes Mom panicked over Dad's behavior, their health, or getting daily tasks accomplished. One morning Mom started crying. Watching her, Dad said, "The only thing I like about all of this is my hat."

"Maybe that's what we need," I told her, "a hat."

"Yes," she agreed, "a hat."

After that, when things became upsetting, we'd say, "We need a hat."

Dad remembered that he had been employed at the steel mill and worried about when to go to work. We would patiently explain that he had been retired for more than twenty years. Though we tried to distract him with another topic, we repeated the same conversation dozens of times.

As the days passed, Dad grew more peaceful and relaxed. When he wasn't out working, he enjoyed looking through the stacks of photo albums, but he didn't understand the concept of photographs. He would smile and coo at the babies as if they were real. Even though it was strange, I felt glad to see him so happy. One picture worried him: a two-year-old grandchild playing in the gravel. Every time he saw that picture, he'd frown and say, "She's going to scrape her legs." One picture was of a grandson throwing a Frisbee. He exclaimed, "Look! He threw it, and it got stuck right in the air!"

After a few days of being home, he could find the bathroom on his own. Once we heard him cry out. Instead of using the toilet, he had begun to take a bath and had turned the water on too hot. After that, we checked on him whenever he went into the bathroom.

Surprisingly, he could still shave, tell time, and read. He liked to read this book about homeless kids. He'd shake his head and ask, "Is this true?" A few minutes later he would read it again and ask the same thing.

Ironically, there were some advantages to his memory loss. He forgot to be grumpy. He forgot that he didn't like to do housework, so he helped Mom around the house. He forgot that it wasn't manly to say "I love you" or to bring Mom roses from the garden.

As the three weeks passed, I kept an eye on Dad, tried to be supportive of Mom, and enjoyed visiting with my youngest sister, Karen. Then it was time to return to Nebraska.

In Ohio, our plane's departure time had been moved up an hour, so we missed the plane. When we arrived in St. Louis for a very short layover, two airport employees pushed Mom and Dad in wheelchairs as we raced across the airport. My parents were a few steps ahead of me when they began to board the plane. Dad stumbled on the uneven ramp and fell. After he got up, everyone kept asking him if he was okay.

"I'm fine. I'm fine," he repeated. Finally, in exasperation he said, "Look! I can walk. I can run. I can chase lions!"

"Yep, he's fine," I said.

In the women's restroom at the Lincoln airport, he stopped at a mirror to chat with his reflection. As we left, he said, "That was a nice fella in there." I had to agree.

Though we had some crazy times together during those days, which would be the last my parents spent in their home, I caught several glimpses of the old Dad. As I observed his warmth, his sense of humor, and his love for hard work, I discovered that regardless of his strange behavior, I still enjoyed being with him. Even though he wasn't like he used to be, Dad was still Dad—that really nice fella who could chase lions.

—*Connie L. Peters*

The Connection

"She'll be so happy to see you all!" I say with as much enthusiasm as I can muster.

In the back of my mind, I know she won't even recognize us. I think to myself that she would have loved my kids so much if she were well. Every once in a while, I see a glimmer in her eyes that reveals an "aha" moment: *Yes, I know these people, but from when, where, how?* Sometimes, I convince myself that this visit will be different, that she'll remember me and we'll leave off just where we were years ago. At the least, I hope that when we visit she'll be happy and full of joy to see us, even if we are perfect strangers to her now. Most of the time, though, I leave the nursing home near tears, unable to accept that this has happened to her. When I am home, I get the urge to call her just to chat, but I know I can't. Every day, with every turn, I miss my dearest friend.

"Jake, please hold Mallory's hand while I carry Rachel, okay?"

I look at my little man of three and a half years and realize that my children would follow me into a fire. That feeling is familiar to me; it is what has brought me here to visit the person I've trusted most in my life. But all that's left of the life-giving fire that once burned inside her is a cooling ember. It is painful to see the light dim on this spitfire—a woman who was always very alive, dancing the jig, doing windmills and sit-ups before bed, and walking faster than me on the beach because she always had a direction in life. She is my grandma, the one person in my universe who loved me unconditionally and who made me feel smart, sweet, and capable of all things. She was the one constant in my life, the one who played with me and laughed with me and taught me. She taught me so many card games, and she loved to play games until she forgot how.

I open the heavy door, and we enter the air-conditioned nursing home. My two followers edge up closer. For a child, being among old, unknown people is scary. I tell my kids that they are all someone else's grandma or grandpa, hoping they will somehow relax as they follow me. Memories flood my mind as we weave around wheelchairs and medication carts. Grandma taught me that there is beauty in plastic beads as well as in real pearls. She made a big deal out of ordinary things. She even made washing dishes fun.

We finally arrive at the door of Grandma's room, and I hope it is a good day as we walk in. Grandma is pacing in front of the window, wringing her hands. Her clothes are the same as on my last visit: pink polyester pants and a floral smock. Pictures of family members cover the walls. I wonder if she looks at them.

"Hi, Grandma," I say. "Come over and sit down. Look who I brought to see you."

She looks startled and then distant. After laying my infant daughter, Rachel, on the colorful afghan, handmade by Grandma, on the bed, I have a free hand to guide my grandmother over to the chair. Her silver hair is brushed back behind her ears; her eyes are still the bluest blue I've ever seen.

I sit on the bed next to Rachel; Jake and Mallory stand close to me at first and then wander around the room while I "chat" with Grandma. I have to do all the talking, and I try to make it as easy as possible for my kids. "Look at how big Jake is now." . . . "Isn't Mallory's hair long?" . . . "Do you remember my last visit, when I was ready to pop?"

Grandma is actually looking at my children, taking them all in, one by one. I coax Mallory into sharing some Sunday school songs. She sings "Jesus Loves Me" in her quiet, bashful beautifulness. This is hard stuff, but I can't break down and cry, although I certainly want to. I want to scream at the heavens. Meanwhile, Grandma smiles and seems to sway to the tune. My mood lightens just to see her smile.

I start singing "Frère Jacques," and Jake and Mallory join in. Grandma probably sang this with me a hundred times before, and she sings a little bit with my kids and me now. This was a favorite of hers, and she would always tell me how, when she was a girl, she'd taken French and Latin in high school.

Because of my grandmother, I, too, learned to enjoy school. I admired her unique handwriting; I was surprised to learn that when she was in school, they actually had a handwriting class. Grandma helped me practice my handwriting in the second grade. She was my guiding light in so many ways. I still carry with me many of her sayings and life lessons: "Nice girls blot." "Pretty is as pretty does." "Beans, beans, the musical fruit, the more you eat the more you toot!"

How can someone be so full of life and laughs one minute become a person with no emotions and no connections virtually the next? How can a wonderful mother, aunt, grandmother, sister, wife, and friend become so unreachable?

Jake is nearly out the door, flirting with the nice nurses and aides, so I know our visit must draw to a close. I'm running out of things to say and growing weary of our one-way conversation. Now, I've reached the point in the visit when I'm just grappling at anything to feel my grandma the way I once knew her. The smiles and the singing have been very sweet, and I know God has blessed me with this little bit. Yet, I want more.

Family had been everything to Grandma, and to her, all babies were precious. This is the first time I've been to the nursing home since Rachel's birth. She'll be a newborn for such a short time, and I want my grandmother to touch her, to hold her.

"Grandma, would you like to hold Rachel?"

The look in her eyes is one of fear and yearning at the same time. No words are expressed. She looks down at her hands as though she is questioning her capabilities. I carefully lay my four-week infant in her receiving arms. I watch my grandmother very closely, ready to sweep Rachel up at the slightest hint she might be dropped. But Grandma is holding my daughter with great care, with the competence of someone who has held many babies. A connection: she remembers being a grandma. I feel as though she remembers holding me.

"Isn't she beautiful?" I say softly.

Grandma looks into my face. She has tears in her eyes.

—*Christine Kiley*

Sand

The sand is relentless. When we visit my parents at their house on Lake Michigan, it pours out of our shoes and spills from our swimsuits at night. It filters down through the rugs on the floor. We brush it vigorously from the sheets before climbing into bed.

Dad tackles it as he does most things: steadily and patiently. He doesn't impose warnings or techniques for prevention on us—his four children, our spouses, and the grandchildren who are visiting. He appreciates the difficulties of sand. The beach is practically right outside the door, after all, and we are in and out of the house all day long.

He routinely starts with the kitchen. He sweeps the wooden floor and takes the rugs outside. He picks up jogging shoes, flip-flops, and tiny yellow sandals. He empties each one and sets it back with the other pairs. He throws the socks and wet towels down the basement stairs, where the washing machine lives.

It helps to have routines if you are tackling sand every day, or if, like my dad, you have early Alzheimer's. He asks the same question twice in a row or mentions a band concert he'd like to see three times in ten minutes. The other day he forgot to bring the boat keys to the marina. He loses things: his wallet, his glasses, his hat. Routines cut down on loss. It helps if you place your keys in the same basket when you come home and always keep your sunglasses on the dashboard in the car. Routines also cut down on stress.

At first, before we could put a name to what was happening, my dad's forgetfulness created a great deal of stress in our family, especially for my mother, who kept insisting something was wrong. We children denied that anything was amiss, some of us more than others, and some quite vigorously, even blaming my mother for overreacting or imagining things. But now, a few years later—after reviewing test results from the University of Michigan, where he takes part in a research study about memory loss and aging, and after meeting with his doctor—we more or less accept what has happened. Now we tend to hear what he does remember, rather than what he doesn't, and to feel grateful for each remembered thing.

It falls on my mother to help him remember. She whispers the name of the woman approaching them at church coffee hour, answers his questions two and three times, and repeats the day's schedule. Sometimes she loses her patience with it. She is afraid it will get worse and worries about what will happen if something happens to her too.

Dad has always been good at following daily routines. He swims in the lake and jogs to the pier, which keeps him trim and physically fit. He and my mother never miss their nightly Scrabble game. When we were growing up, Dad woke at 5:30 every morning of the week. He went to work, where he performed delicate surgery on the inner ear, and taught medical students at the University of Michigan, a job he loved. At home he built tree forts in our yard and hung a trapeze in the basement. My brother said he sometimes closes his eyes tight and wills himself to remember what Dad was like when we were little, all the things he did for us.

The youngest grandchild, Kaia, patient and still like her grandfather, tries to dig a hole in the sand on the beach. With each scoop, more sand falls in. The older kids regale my parents with this story. "Kaia digs a hole like this!" her fast-talking, ten-year-old sister, Madeline, says, pantomiming the scoop of the shovel and then fluttering her fingers to show the sand falling back in. Scoop, flutter, scoop, flutter. It seems so futile.

The sand will continue to come inside the house as long as we venture out—to the beach, to the woods, to the lake. Yet, there is a moment, right after the house is swept, when Dad appears to have it conquered. The house doesn't look terribly different; it's the way it feels, smooth and solid underfoot. It is reassuring just knowing that he persists, that he has swept the sand out one more time.

—Lydie Raschka

Doing Our Best

A tight fist struck the dining table with such force that the table shook.

It was my eighty-year-old mother's fist, and it landed directly in front of her eighty-six-year-old roommate sitting across from her. Mother needed to make a point, one she'd probably wanted to make for months, but until that moment, she hadn't been able to bring the thought and the action together. As though the blow to the table were not enough, she simultaneously shouted, "Put a sock in it!"

I wasn't there to witness this scene, but, my daughter, Christina, was. She said she'd been stunned but then had to choke back a giggle. My feelings were also mixed. I felt bad for Lucy that Mother had behaved that way, yet I was honestly thrilled to know that she had succeeded in verbally expressing what she was feeling. For such a long time, I'd watched her struggle to put words together—to ask or answer questions, to simply say whatever was on her mind. Now, she'd not only managed to speak her mind, but her words had formed a full sentence.

Sadly, both my mother and Lucy suffered from Alzheimer's. Mother was persistent in her efforts to speak; Lucy, on the other hand, couldn't talk at all. She just made a lot of noise. Actually, she made only one repetitive sound that increased in volume each time it escaped her mouth. This occurred intermittently throughout the day. Some nights she would do it in her sleep, and that was a double whammy for Mother. A large dressing table was all that separated their beds. The caregivers did their best to quiet Lucy, and most of the time, the other residents appeared to simply tune her out. Nonetheless, it wasn't easy for anyone, including Lucy, I'm sure, and especially for my mother.

Mother lived in the home of a wonderful family who took care of five residents diagnosed with Alzheimer's. The home was conveniently located between my office and my home. So, normally, I was able to go by and spend at least an hour or two with my mother before her bedtime. Lucy's noises were only one of the many things that were strange and new to my mother. It was understandable that it would take time for her to adjust. I felt sure the transition would be easier for her if I could see her on a daily basis, but one week I was exceptionally busy at work, so for three days straight I was unable to visit Mother.

As I drove to see her on Thursday, I couldn't shake the questions troubling my mind: *Had Mother wondered where I was? Was she upset, or feeling abandoned?* I knew her caregiver, Nellie, had explained my absence, but I was still not at peace. Mentally, Mother lived in a different world now, and it was often difficult to be certain of how much she understood or remembered. In addition to the effects of Alzheimer's, she was living in a new house, city, and state, none of which she recognized, and I felt sure she was confused and even frightened. I knew I was frightened. In fact, I felt helpless in many ways, but I believed that it had been a wise decision to move her from Texas to California. At least now I could spend more time with her and monitor her evolving health issues.

Mother's condition had crept up on both of us but mostly me. She had long suspected the possibility of having Alzheimer's, but she didn't share her fears with anyone, except to say how frustrated she was by her forgetfulness. She had a lot of tension in her life, so I initially thought the forgetfulness was a combination of stress and aging. When I was moving her, however, I discovered she'd been researching the disease. In drawers and boxes I found pamphlets she'd ordered through the mail and articles cut from magazines and newspapers.

Personality changes had developed slowly. During visits and phone conversations, I had noticed she'd become short-tempered. The next change that puzzled me was the paranoia; she hid personal items, thinking someone wanted to steal them. The short-term memory loss seemed natural, but when my aunt said Mother had been getting lost enroute to places she'd driven to for years, I became alarmed. After a fall in which she sustained serious injuries, I was convinced she needed twenty-four-hour care.

Nellie's home came highly recommended, but I was extremely hesitant to trust anyone to take care of my mother. After meeting the family and after seeing the immaculately clean, well-organized house, I began to relax. We discussed Mother's condition and needs at great length, and I realized I couldn't manage on my own.

"Sherry," Nellie said, "I know how difficult this is, but I promise to take care of your mother as though she were my own."

Though I'd just met this pretty, petite woman with her amazing, infectious smile, I sensed very quickly that I could trust her.

My instincts about Nellie and her home proved to be accurate, but I was still faced with the reality that even with the best of care, my mother's condition would gradually deteriorate. I could never be sure what to expect from day to day, but one amazing thing I was always certain of was that Mother never failed to recognize me and my daughter, Christina.

Whenever she saw us, her face lit up with an ear-to-ear smile and her eyes danced with pleasure. We talked to her about everything, just as we always had. During her last two years, she began to respond through body language more than with words. She would listen, her eyes glued to ours, and nod her head, occasionally speaking the best she could. We had learned how to make Mother feel comfortable with her limited means of communication. She seemed convinced that we always understood her. I learned to expect both good days and bad. Through it all, I truly believed that Mother's mind was not totally lost—just often misplaced.

A few weeks after the "fist" incident, I witnessed another less noisy, but cherished moment. It was during my first visit after I'd not been by for three days.

I hurried into Nellie's family room, where Mother was sitting in her usual spot on a green, leather sofa, her favorite flowered throw pillow propped behind her head. As I crossed the room, I thought to myself, *She looks smaller and frailer.* I sat beside her and positioned myself so we were face to face.

"Mommy," I said, "I've been working longer hours. I'm so sorry I haven't been over, but I didn't want to come late and wake you." As my words spilled out and ran together, I obviously looked as anxious and worried as I felt and sounded.

Looking concerned but calm, Mother reached out, grasped my hands, and holding them in her lap, she said, "Its okay, baby, I know you do your best."

Thank you, Lord, I thought, *another complete and coherent sentence.*

I rested my head in that comfortable little nook between my mother's neck and shoulder. I didn't want her to see my tears. I'd shed many tears of sadness since learning she had Alzheimer's. This time they were tears of joy. It had been so long since she'd seemed like the mother I'd known: always there for me, ready to listen, and always understanding. Over the years, she sometimes didn't like the choices I made, but I could always count on Mother to stand by me. Now, after struggling with the realization that this dreadful disease was gradually taking her away, I felt certain that wherever her mind was at any given time, she kept me with her.

Since my childhood, Mother had always said to me, "All I ask is that you do your best." Those words meant more to me that day than ever before. Somehow, she understood that I hadn't been by for a while, but she also knew I'd done what she'd always asked of me—my best.

During one of my daughter's visits with my mother, they were sitting at the dining table together, where Christina was telling her grandmother about something that had happened on campus that day. Her story was met with a blank stare. Christina repeated herself, but still got no response.

"Mum, did you hear what I said?" she asked.

Angelina, another resident, was sitting at the end of the table having a snack. She had lived at Nellie's for almost a year. Although we'd occasionally heard this delightful little Italian woman quietly mumble a few words to no one in particular, she had never spoken in English. She had obviously been listening to Christina, because she suddenly looked at her and clearly said, "Go ahead and tell her about it, honey. We understand."

Christina called me as soon as she left Nellie's. "Mom," she excitedly exclaimed, "Angelina spoke, and she told me, in English, that they do understand what we say."

Times like those were what kept our hopes alive. I was sure Mother understood that her life had changed drastically, but she couldn't understand why. She did live in her own world, but somehow she kept a foot in ours.

She was so happy when we took her out for pizza or ice cream. Sometimes, those outings were a struggle for her and for us, particularly when the disease began to affect her motor skills. It was difficult for her to get in and out of the car. Going up and down steps was also a problem, and eventually I was lifting her feet one at a time, step by step. I would say to her, "There's no hurry, Mommy. I know you're doing your best." And she was. It was as though her mind and heart were at war, and her heart won. She wouldn't give up, because we wouldn't give up.

But her body had a say as well, and it grew tired of fighting. Mother had a stroke. I brought her to my house, where she lived her last two weeks. My sister came from Florida, and she, Christina, and I sat on or beside Mother's bed around the clock.

I had come to believe that at any stage of the disease, a person with Alzheimer's could feel love in the deepest level of their consciousness. We expressed our love through touch, massaging her beautiful body in hopes of making her more comfortable. We talked to her, reminiscing about times past, the present, and the future. We assured her that we'd be with her again one day, and that, meanwhile, we would take good care of each other. Finally, with great difficulty, we gave her permission to let go. We knew she needed to hear those words before she could leave us.

When she left, we were holding her. It was the very best we could do.

—Sherry Matthews

Loss, Love, and Acceptance

"**T**he bathroom is on the right, Mom."

"Here?"

"No, the other way."

"This way?"

"No, turn a little bit more."

"This way?"

"Almost." I got up and gently rotated her shoulders and pointed to the bathroom entrance.

"That's it. Okay!"

Phew! I sighed. We were two days into my mother's planned thirty-day winter visit to our home. Her Alzheimer's condition had worsened since the last stay. We were still working on finding the bathroom.

I struggled to accept my caretaking role. All of my adult life I had ached for my mother to visit me as I traveled with my husband from one military post to another, but she had never felt she could break free of her many responsibilities to come and simply have fun. I felt cheated now, because our time would be colored by a debilitating disease instead of being the joyous sharing I had always imagined. Still, I was determined to have my special time with her. Today I had planned a fun day of gazing at exotic fish in the National Aquarium, shopping, watching ice-skaters, and eating at fine restaurants.

As it turned out, however, the subtitle for all of this hoped-for frivolity proved to be "Mom's teeth." In the gift shop she took out her false teeth because she had a piece of caramel stuck in them. It took us an hour to scrape it off. Then later, at the Hyatt Restaurant, I followed the horrified gaze of our server to discover Mom washing her teeth in the water pitcher. Making a hurried exit and attempting to redirect her attention, we posed for pictures after asking a strange man to hold my camera.

"Sex!" Mom yelled, grinning mischievously as the flash exploded. I mumbled a sheepish "thank you" and retrieved our camera as we scurried away from the astonished gentleman. I felt exhausted and humbled, not to mention just plain adrift in uncharted waters.

Mother had always been my port in a storm, my guru, my model of competence and efficiency. At every stage of my life she had guided me through the growth issues important to thriving. Comfort, safety, love: the early years. Encouragement, patience, praise: the pre-adolescent years.

"You can do anything you can visualize," she would say, "anything you can set your mind to."

And I believed her. I achieved successes in school and in extracurricular activities that caused others to assume I was gifted and talented. But I wasn't. I simply followed excellent advice given by a master. In my teen years, Mom listened and listened and listened. In my college years, she trusted me implicitly, aided me concretely, and communicated frequently. As the grandmother of my children, she loved them unconditionally and joyfully.

My mother's heart, mind, and hands worked in perfect harmony as she brought forth her best to those around her. She showed me by example how to serve my family, my friends, and my community. When I was growing up, we were, by any standards, financially poor, but I didn't realize it until I looked back on my childhood as a more affluent adult. My mother hadn't indulged in self-pity, and she wouldn't allow her daughters to, either. Gratitude was to be our attitude. After all, just look at all we had to be thankful for.

There's a family photo of my sister and me taken in our dusty yard, the west Texas sun and wind competing for dominance. We are scrubbed clean, standing straight, and flashing huge smiles. Our homemade dresses are pressed, and our hair shines in the bright sun. We look pleased with ourselves, as happy children do when posing for a picture. I know now that the only difference between us and the poignant photographs of dirty Depression-era children staring blankly through fences was the love, faith, skill, and determination of our mother.

Now in my middle age, when I trusted my mother to show me how to transition to the next stage of life—how to age gracefully, how to live my elder years with courage, insight, and meaning—it was my task to show her the bathroom and to shield her from astonished, gaping strangers. *How could this be? Hadn't my grandmother and great-grandmother lived to become the "wise women" of their communities, dispensing love and advice well into their nineties? Hadn't Mom earned the right to be their heir? Where was justice?* I railed. *Where was peace? Where*, I finally asked, *was God?*

Like most of humanity through the ages, I received no clear-cut answers. I simply had to keep trying to muddle through.

What activities can be planned with a physically healthy but mentally incompetent seventy-four-year-old woman? We could not talk about the past. Realizing she didn't remember disturbed her. I couldn't discuss my questions about aging or even plans for the future. She merely looked at me blankly. Within an hour she wouldn't be able to remember anything we'd said. I felt frustrated at having the past and the future inaccessible. At the same time, I became aware of how much consciousness I had been devoting to those illusory worlds.

Mom still knew who I was, thank goodness, and we could share the warmth of affectionate touches and the intimacy of eye contact. I quickly learned to plan things one step at a time, since multitasking was impossible. The combination yielded surprising results. We walked for hours along beautiful nature trails and gloried in the sun on our faces, squealing if we saw a deer or a rabbit. How tasty food became. How beautiful the colors around us. How sublime the music we played on a quiet evening. The words "hot tub" defined sensual delight. Occasionally, we would roll our eyes, sigh, and giggle like teenagers at the sight of a great male physique walking away from us. I began to experience what Zen masters call the "eternal now."

Nothing prepared me, however, for the sudden change that occurred two weeks into the visit. I woke up one morning to find Mom clumsily packing her suitcase. "I want to go home," she said, throwing personal items into her bag without any attention to organizing.

At first I thought something had happened to upset her. "What's wrong?" I asked softly, walking toward her. "I'm looking forward to the next two weeks." I tried to touch her on the shoulder, but she jerked away and looked at me quizzically.

"I want to go home!" she wailed defiantly. "Cindy is my life. I feel as though I am her. Don't keep me here. You can't make me stay!"

I couldn't believe it. My mother was acting like a rebellious teenager. But worse than that, she had lost control over her emotions and let me know that my sister, her primary caretaker now, was her favorite. I was stunned, embarrassed for her, and sorry for myself. I needed time to think—time to get my own feelings back under control.

"I have a headache," I lied, as I headed down the hall. "I need to rest a few minutes. I'll be out soon. Okay?"

She looked at me like a child who has no other choice.

"Okay," she mouthed softly, closing her lips in a thin, pouting line and crossing her arms in front of her. She looked away, as tears formed.

I battled long-suppressed demons in the safety of my bedroom. I thought of all those times she had refused to visit me, times I had been so homesick. My alcoholic father would not let her come, she would explain. Or my grandmother was ill and needed her. It was always something. I had reluctantly believed her. But now I wondered, *What did all that mean? Were those merely excuses? She really didn't like being with me at all?* I sobbed into a pillow as suppressed pain from the past met the raw grief of the present.

Eventually, I spent my tears and slipped into a breathing meditation. Then half-dozing, I allowed early memories to quietly enter my consciousness. My first memory was of our bedroom—Daddy's, Mama's, and mine. I remember where my bed stood and how I stood in it. The floors were concrete, and later I learned to love the cold against my bare feet. I could hear the screen door open and close and the sounds from the neighborhood surrounding it. Sometimes the screen door opened to other tears, Mama's tears. We had a silver butane tank that I pretended was my horse and a green wooden picnic table, where birthday cakes were served and where Mama quietly cried in the twilight when I was very young. Supposedly, when my older sister was three, Mama tied her to that table to keep her from running away while I was being bathed. But my sister's rebellion did not cause the tears I saw from my room. No, they were the grief of dreams lost and an acknowledgement of a life much harder than planned.

Yet, Mother had matured into a patient and kind woman, finally learning to love everyone unconditionally. I had watched her change and grow from a frustrated young mother into a wise and centered woman. No one had ever celebrated my mother's life to my liking, and now even I was among those who always wanted to be on the receiving end of her affection. Could I also learn to love unconditionally? I dried my own tears of loss and acceptance, and I went to her.

"Okay, okay." I soothed her gently. "I'll let you go, I promise. Not today, but soon. Everything will be all right."

She relaxed. We hugged.

I didn't realize then that I had, indeed, let her go or that we had hugged good-bye. The next morning when I awoke, she was sitting in a chair beside our bed, humming softly.

"Swing low, sweet chariot, comin' for to carry me home . . ." When she saw me sitting up, she stared for a long moment, wide-eyed. "Who are you?" she asked. "Who are you?"

And with that final question, my mother had once again given me everything I needed to go on.

—S. Ann Robinson

My Mother's House

The call came late one evening when I was nearly three hours from home, driving up north to a weekend retreat. I fumbled for my cell phone, and my heart sank when I saw the display flash the number for my mother's caregiving service. I pulled over to the side of the road and answered.

"A bad fall . . . We're at the hospital . . . Her hip . . ."

I clutched my steering wheel and began madly to figure out logistics, trying to ignore my growing feeling of alarm. *When could I get back? How would I reach my sister and my husband? What should I tell my daughter, who was camping with a friend?*

Overarching everything was worry about what my mother was feeling, in her narrow and increasingly puzzling world. The caregiver had said she was not yet alarmed or agitated; perhaps if we got a familiar face there quickly enough, it would keep her calm and focused while the hospital tended to her.

I spent most of the night on the telephone, sitting cross-legged on the bed in my retreat cabin, my suitcase still packed, trying to keep abreast of what was happening at home. My sister and my husband had both managed to get to the emergency room to sit with my mother, and it seemed to be helping. As the night wore on and she became more fatigued, however, it became increasingly difficult to reassure her.

The hospital confirmed our fears. My mother's hip was broken and she was admitted to the orthopedic unit. She was not in a lot of pain, but she was baffled as to why she was in the hospital, forgetting she had been injured, asking after her little girls, wanting to go home. My sister, Judy, had stayed there with her, but Judy needed me to come home as quickly as I could get away. Things were very hectic, and there was much to handle, with the battery of tests and needles and X-rays and medications and with my mother's growing confusion and consternation.

As I roared south the next morning, I lamented the timing that had caused me to be so far away during this crisis. Each time I left town, I dreaded leaving my mother. I worried that the caretaker might get sick and not report for work. I fretted about her medications and her safety. I imagined her watching in vain out the window, always waiting for us to come home for supper, the daughters who had moved out of her home more than three decades ago.

The surgery to repair my mother's broken hip left Judy and me drained and my mother disoriented and sobbing. We bent over her, reassuring her, caressing her hand, telling her she was safe.

"I want to go home," she whimpered. "I feel as if I am in a horrible place. Everyone is a stranger. I want to go home."

No matter how many times we reminded her, she could not remember her fall, even with the pain in her hip. She asked repeatedly where she was, tried to get out of bed, tore out her IV, and took off her surgical dressing. The hospital set up a bed in my mother's room, and Judy and I took shifts staying with her, trying to keep her grounded and centered as best we could in frightening surroundings.

While Judy took the first turn watching over our mother, I went to Mom's house to pick up some of her things. I sat alone in the living room, gazing around me and wanting nothing more than to slump over on the couch and wail with sorrow. The house breathed my mother: her things, her voice, her footsteps. I remembered sitting so often in just this spot on the couch, her slender body close to mine. She would hold my hand, rubbing my fingers.

"Why, your little paddies are cold, honey!" she would sometimes say, stretching out her skirt to cover my legs, tucking the folds across my knees.

My mother's struggle with dementia had not yet altered the inherent sweetness of her character, and we prayed to be spared that aspect of Alzheimer's. We were blessed that the progression of her disease had been gradual, and we had fought to keep her in her own home as her world became more and more bewildering to her, believing that she found a certain anchor in a familiar environment and in the presence of her old dog, Sam. *What if she could not return here?* I fretted now. *What if this accident was the turning point that would open a new phase in her, and our, lives?*

Along with those worries, another more selfish thought loomed in my mind: I was frightened by the idea of her living elsewhere. This was my mother's house, the place where she had lived for nearly sixty years. This was where I was born, where my sister was born, where we had played and grown up, where I had lived while I was in college, where our pets were buried, where my father spent his last years, and where I pictured my mother in every room, every corner of the house. This was where she was. When I was here with her in this house, I could occasionally pretend time had stopped. Sometimes I could even imagine she was not ill.

Over the next two weeks, Judy or I stayed with my mother all of the time she was in the hospital, reassuring her, entertaining her with word puzzles and photos, talking to her, bringing her little presents. She was on her feet within two days and walked down the hall with the help of an aide and a walker, an accomplishment that astonished the hospital staff and put a germ of hope in a secret corner of my heart. I just wanted to get her home, to get her back to where things were before the accident occurred.

Sometimes my mother was lucid and reasonable during her hospital stay; sometimes she became angry at being restrained and with her inability to force her body—until then amazingly strong for an eighty-six-year-old woman—to do the things she felt it should be able to do.

Judy and I shared our worries with each other, did our best to remain patient, and carried on, trying not to agonize about the future. Or at least I believe Judy tried. For my part, at the first opportunity I went back to my mother's house and sat alone in the silence, obsessing about turning back the clock, remembering what it was like when we had seen the first clues of her disorientation. Forgotten names, forgotten dates, out-of-place comments, uncharacteristic displays of emotion—those problems had intensified over the years and now were spotlighted with this stay in the hospital. *If only I could get her home,*

I thought for the millionth time. *If only this could be just a temporary bump in the road.*

I looked at the piles of the crossword books she loved and at the charity mail she always opened and set aside to consider later (and which we usually quietly spirited away). There was her afghan—the place where she took her naps, where she sat to read, often the same chapter over and over again. Her bedroom slippers sat neatly by her bed. And there were her coffee cup, her eyebrow pencil, and her toothpaste, carefully rolled from the bottom. Her things, these remnants of her life, were everywhere. I wanted my mother back—here, where she belonged.

We soldiered on, and finally, we were able to move her to a rehab facility. As we carried piles of her things inside, I felt my heart growing somber and the beginnings of panic. The future was still in question, and she looked so right in her small room, with her belongings around her—photos of Sam and of us, her own clothing hung in the closet.

I watched her move laboriously from her chair to the bed, and I went to sit by her, wanting just to be near her, to soak up the comfort of her presence. We sat there in silence for a moment, and then she took my hand.

"Why, your little paddies are cold, honey!" she said, and pulled the edge of her sweater across my shoulders.

—Loraine J. Hudson

Close Call

Amanda sat in her favorite chintz armchair and wished for a means of escape. The telephone resting on the inlaid oak end table mocked her with its promise of easy accessibility. She thought of the old slogan, "Reach out and touch someone." If only she still could. Tears slipped down her cheeks as she summoned the courage to pick up the phone. A simple act, but one that had become increasingly difficult as the months passed. *Just make the call.* Amanda's thoughts seemed to echo in the empty living room; her family accepted her need to face this weekly ordeal in private. *She probably won't answer. Oh, just make the call and be done with it.*

For years Amanda had looked forward to her weekly chats with her mother, an opportunity to sweep away the intervening miles and to share small but precious details of their lives. Now, that simple joy had turned into a trial. A vortex of early memories imprisoned Amanda's mother, holding her captive within her own mind. Her recent history wavered in confused disarray. The present? Completely unintelligible.

Amanda counted as her mom's phone rang: six . . . seven . . . eight . . . nine (almost there; she gave herself permission to hang up after ten) . . . ten.

"Hello?" The feeble voice registered in Amanda's consciousness just before she disconnected. "Who's there?"

"Good morning, Mom. It's Amanda." She forced a cheerful note into her words. "Are you having a nice day?"

"Who?" Mom paused, and Amanda imagined her, white-haired and frail, staring out the wide picture window that occupied one wall of her room in the nursing home half a continent away in Kansas. "Oh, Rachel! It's so good to hear from you. I've been worried about little Peter."

Amanda sighed. For the moment, it seemed Amanda was Aunt Rachel, Mom's older sister, dead five years.

"Don't worry about Peter. He's doing just fine," Amanda said. "Tell me about your flowers." Sometimes she could pull her mom closer to the present by talking about the flower arrangement Amanda sent every Friday.

"Oh, they're just beautiful this year. The roses are climbing so high we can barely see through the kitchen window."

Time to try again. "Mom, this is Amanda . . . your daughter."

"Well, I know who you are!" Exasperation edged Mom's voice. "Why would you think I didn't?"

"Never mind. I just wanted to tell you I love you." The lump in her throat expanded, and Amanda fought to keep her tone light. She took a deep breath and swallowed her grief. Her mother might not remember the year or that she had children, grandchildren, and great-grandchildren, but she picked up on emotions like a finely tuned receiver. If Amanda choked up, her mom would be overcome with her own volatile emotions. The hardworking nursing home staff deserved better than that.

"That's nice, dear." Her voice sounded distant, as if the telephone reception were fading. "Did I tell you I'm getting an apartment closer to town?"

Amanda closed her eyes and let the familiar litany wash over her. Life would be so much easier once her mom moved to the imagined apartment; she'd be closer to the college she'd never attended. Amanda rubbed her aching temples. At least her mom was active and happy in her alternate reality.

Why did she bother with these weekly calls? Why did she torture herself this way? Her mom didn't benefit; she forgot the call as soon as it ended, and rarely did she realize who was actually on the other end of the line. The calls certainly didn't benefit Amanda. The inability to communicate left her dangling helplessly between two poles. She ached to mourn, but to do so while her mother was alive reeked of disloyalty.

During the week, Amanda could allow her mom's condition to slip from her consciousness. But her subconscious never forgot. It heaped abuse on her because she wasn't there, wasn't caring for her mother personally. And Amanda probed that wound every Saturday morning. Perhaps the weekly bloodletting served a purpose, allowing the poisons of self-abuse to drain as she again realized her inability to deal with the mother who was no longer her mother. All she knew for sure was that the calls left her drained and empty.

"You know, Amanda, what can't be cured must be endured."

Amanda gasped, yanked from her bleak thoughts by the vitality in her mom's voice.

"What did you say?"

"You heard me, sweetheart," she said. Her voice, strong and vibrant with love, amazed Amanda. "Just remember your quilts. If all the fabric is beautiful, the quilt is boring. It's the uglies that give it life, that make the design sing."

"Oh, Mom! I've missed you so much." The emotional dam dissolved and tears streamed across Amanda's cheeks. She wanted to cram information through the phone—to rejoice with her mom about her infant grandson, to tell her about the new house, its gardens a riot of color and texture—but the knot in her throat choked the words.

"I know you have." Her mother's voice sounded strangled as well. "Always remember, I love you with all my heart."

Amanda grabbed a tissue, blew her stuffy nose, and said, "I know you do, Mom."

"Do what?" The petulant whine had returned to the other end of the line. "Who is this? Why are you bothering me?"

"It's Amanda, Mom. I just called to say I love you."

—Debbie Mumford

Names have been changed to protect the privacy of the people in this story and their loved ones.

Apple, Hat, Ashtray

When my mother called to say that the neurologist wanted all of us at Dad's next appointment, my heart sank. For months, he'd been having trouble with forgetfulness, confusion, and was having outright bizarre behavior. He'd been tested for Alzheimer's at least two times, but the diagnosis always came back inconclusive or ruled out Alzheimer's altogether. I knew from Mom's voice that this time was different, but I wanted desperately to cling to a bit of denial.

Dad's older sister had been diagnosed with Alzheimer's five years earlier. Aunt Rosalie had always been considered the beauty of the family. She had piercing blue eyes, wavy auburn hair, and a dazzling smile. Not only was she physically striking, she also possessed the same Irish wit and charm as my father. Even into her seventies, she had a sense of style and personality that drew people to her. In the five years since Aunt Rosalie had been diagnosed, we'd watched her grow at first distant, then incoherent, and then completely withdrawn into a world of dementia from which she never emerged.

Dad's appointment was at a medical building in midtown Kansas City. It was early March, and though the sun was shining as brightly as a spring morning in May, it was cold and blustery. I pulled into a parking space and yanked the collar of my coat up around my neck as I stepped from the car. Sharp wind stung my eyes and flattened strands of hair across my face as I hurried toward the glass doors of the office building.

My parents were already in the lobby, along with my oldest sister, Cecelia, and my younger brother, Patrick. After exchanging hugs and greetings, we boarded the elevator that took us to the eleventh floor. On the way up, I wondered if my brother and sister were also holding on to a bit of denial.

We exited the elevator and followed a gray carpeted hallway to the doctor's suite. The receptionist, a young woman with a thick mane of blonde hair, directed us to a sunny conference room to wait on the neurologist.

He strode into the room right on time. He was tall and balding with rimless glasses perched on the bridge of a prominent nose. He wore a spotless white lab coat over a yellow shirt and a blue striped tie. He extended his arm in a handshake gesture as soon as he crossed the threshold of the door. "I'm Doctor Levinson," he said, smiling and offering his outstretched hand to each of us in turn. We all sat down at a long conference table, and Dr. Levinson began to speak.

"Your mother has been concerned about your dad and his behavior the last few months," he said, looking at my brother, sister, and me. "She feels like something might be wrong with his memory and cognitive functioning. We've conducted some tests to determine what the cause of these memory and sensory problems might be. I thought it would be helpful for the family to be here when we go over the test results."

I felt a shriveling sensation in my stomach and knew that the bit of denial I'd been holding on to was probably about to be met with stark reality.

"First, I want to run some questions by your dad." Dr. Levinson said, and then turned to Dad. "Jerry, I'm going to go through a series of questions with you. There are no right or wrong answers. You don't need to worry about passing or failing. Just answer if you can, but if you can't, that's perfectly fine."

My father nodded, smiling, his blue eyes sparkling in the bright sunlight that streamed through the conference room windows. "Now, I'm going to give you some words to remember before I ask questions. When I've finished with the questions, I'm going to ask you to remember the words I gave you at the very beginning. Are you ready?"

My father chuckled and nodded. "Sure," he said. "Ready as I'll ever be."

Dad was wearing a blue dress shirt and khaki pants. He had removed his cap, an Irish tweed touring hat, when he'd come into the office. His hair was a little mussed, and some snow-white strands floated halo-like above his pink scalp.

"Jerry," Dr. Levinson said, "I want you to remember these three words when I ask you for them later. The words are: apple, hat, ashtray."

My father looked intently into Dr. Levinson's eyes. "Apple, hat, and ashtray?" he asked tentatively.

"Yes," Dr. Levinson replied, "Apple, hat, and ashtray."

The shriveling sensation turned to outright nausea as reality sunk in. The neurologist had gathered us here to demonstrate that Dad's failing memory was more than just normal aging or elderly forgetfulness. He knew that we needed to see what my mother had been observing for months, maybe even years. The words "apple," "hat," and "ashtray" burned themselves into my brain.

Please, Dad, I thought. *Please remember: apple, hat, ashtray.* I projected my thoughts toward my dad as if I could clairvoyantly transfer "apple," "hat," and "ashtray" right into his head. *Dad, think of an apple wearing a hat and sitting in an ashtray. Please, Dad, an apple wearing a hat, sitting in an ashtray.*

I knew it was irrational, silly even, but I hoped beyond reason that by remembering those three words, the Alzheimer's could be held at bay. Maybe it wasn't really happening, after all. If he could remember "apple," "hat," and "ashtray," I could have my father back. For the last years of his life, my dad would know and love me and take care of my mother like he always had. If Dad could remember "apple," "hat," and "ashtray," life would go on normally. He and my mother would continue to live on their little farm, where my daughters had climbed trees, gathered chicken eggs, and learned about the outdoors from a master naturalist, my father.

On any given night, I could still visit and go outside with Dad to look up at the vast blackness of the cosmos. I could point to the star-laden sky and ask, "Dad, what's that constellation?"

"That star shining so bright in the east over there, that's Venus. You can always tell Venus. In the spring and summer, it sparkles so bright in the eastern sky that you can't miss it," he would say. "And there's the

Big Dipper right over there and then the Little Dipper. Look, you can even see the Milky Way on a night like this. And over there, that's Orion; you can see his belt, how it's made up of three little stars. See?"

Growing up on a farm, my dad had learned astronomy the way that people who make their living from understanding the rhythms and the pulse of nature have to. It was not an academic exercise that drove him to study the night sky and the cycles of the moon; it was survival—that, and just plain being there night after night to gaze up at it all and wonder.

Dr. Levinson led Dad through a series of questions, patiently asking who was president, what day was it and what month, which state did he live in, and how many children did he have. Dad knew who was president; he'd been a political junkie for as long as I could remember. He got the number of children right, too, but there were many questions he missed, questions he should have easily known the answers to.

Throughout the question-and-answer session, Dr. Levinson scribbled notes in a pad. Then, he closed the note pad and turned to my father again.

"Jerry, do you remember the words I mentioned at the beginning of our session?"

My father's face was blank, and then he started to frown, trying to remember what it was he was supposed to say.

Apple, hat, ashtray, I again tried desperately to transmit the words into Dad's head, hoping some miraculous act of ESP would take place. *Apple, hat, ashtray, apple, hat, ashtray. Apple, hat, ashtray.*

The room was quiet as Dad continued struggling to conjure up the words he was asked to remember. Finally, he chuckled nervously and waved his hand in defeat.

"That's all right, Jerry," Dr. Levinson said, "Like I told you, there are no right or wrong answers to these questions. You did fine."

Dr. Levinson cleared his throat, and as he began to talk, I felt a lump in my throat swell to the size of a tennis ball and struggled to maintain composure.

"Alzheimer's is a progressive disease," he said, "and each person is different with regard to how fast or how slowly cognitive function diminishes." He continued on, explaining the kind of medication that would be prescribed and recommending that Dad no longer drive a car. He told my mother he had literature for her and asked us if we had any questions.

Any questions? Yes, I had about a million of them, but none that could be answered by a neurologist. *Why was this happening to my father, who had lived his life always trying to do the right thing, the ethical thing, and taught his children to do likewise? Why wasn't there a cure for a disease that was stealing people from their families and robbing victims of the very essence of what made them who they were?* I felt my bit of denial slip away like raindrops sliding off glass.

My siblings and I left the conference room with Dad. Mom was still talking to the doctor and lagged behind. We decided to meet at a nearby restaurant for lunch.

"I'll take Dad and meet you there," I said.

"That's fine," Cecelia said, "Mom can ride with me."

I led Dad out of the building and across the parking lot, helped him into my minivan, made sure his seat belt was secure, and drove to the parking lot exit. Traffic was heavy. We were quiet as I waited for an opportunity to pull out. Finally, a break in the stream of vehicles opened up, and I darted in. As we headed toward the restaurant, I asked, "Dad, are you scared?"

He looked at me with a puzzled expression. His hat was cocked at a tilt, and tufts of silvery hair poked out around his ears. Like Aunt Rosalie, Dad's age hadn't diminished his good looks or made him any less charming. "Scared? I ain't scared of nothin'!" He laughed, making a joke of it, then reached over and patted my shoulder. "What good would it do to be scared?" he said, his face now serious. "There isn't anything that can be done to change this."

When I pulled up to a stoplight, he turned to me, his blue eyes as solemn as I'd ever seen. "Listen. Kathleen, everything will be okay. You remember that."

"I will, Dad," I said. "I love you."

"I love you, too," he said, giving me another pat on the shoulder.

In the years that followed, I held onto those words, knowing how important it was for him, even while teetering on the brink of losing his own mind, to make sure that I didn't worry or get frightened. It's the kind of father he was. If I honored his desire to protect his family from fear, maybe there was at least one thing that Alzheimer's could not steal from us. "Everything will be okay," became a kind of mantra for me as I watched Dad slip further and further into the depths of dementia.

Sometimes, I think back to that moment when the words "apple," "hat," and "ashtray" seemed so terribly important. At the time, it felt as if the whole universe hung on Dad's ability to pull those words from his memory. Instead, they turned out to be the least important words spoken that day.

—*Kathleen McKenzie-Winn*

Where Are We Going?

The third time eggs exploded all over the kitchen I thought that maybe, just maybe, Mom shouldn't be living by herself anymore. Of course, denial is strong. She's okay, I told myself, just a little forgetful. But I came to learn that Alzheimer's is a slow and unrelenting disease. The signs that all was not well came more and more frequently and with increasing seriousness.

In the beginning, only a person who knew my mother well would have known that something was just not right. After all, who doesn't forget where they put their keys? Who doesn't forget someone's name? But when you are expecting a long-deceased relative to come to dinner, there is something definitely off.

When I think back, I realize that her car accident marked the start of her difficulties. She missed a turn while going home after visiting me. Her car was totaled, some trees lost their bark, and someone's very pretty rock garden was destroyed, but she came out of it without a scratch. She was very lucky that she hadn't hurt herself or someone else. I was glad that the policeman had taken her license away, because I was fully prepared to stop her from driving. Unfortunately, "the very nice policeman" came by her house to return the license and to see how she was. Before I could blink, she had a new car and was driving again.

The next step in the progression was simple. Now the short-term memory loss was accompanied by confusion about places and events that, normally, were very familiar to her. At that point, according to Mom, we were the same age.

"How old are you?" she asked while we were driving.

"I'm sixty."

"Oh, me too."

"You mean, we are the same age, but you're my mother?"

"Yes."

She would forget where she was going or how to get home. I wouldn't learn of these events until something would come up in conversation.

"I went down the street the wrong way, and people were driving at me, honking and waving. I stopped in a parking lot, and a very nice man came and asked me if I was okay. I told him I was fine but that they had changed the road and I got confused. He told me I did some great driving." She said this with pride to prove to me that her driving was just fine. The road had not been changed in twenty years. And we're talking about a major highway.

I never told her that she couldn't drive. However, she lived alone, so she was always glad to have company. It got to be a routine: I would call and ask her if she wanted to come with me to the store, and she would agree. If she told me she was going to take the car to do something, I would suggest we do it together. She is not stupid. She caught on and went along with it. I believe that she was scared to drive but too stubborn to admit it.

By then, her short-term memory was almost non-existent. "Where are we going?" became her mantra.

"We're going to the store, Mom."

"Oh." Silence. Two minutes later: "Where are we going?"

We had settled the driving problem, but now the fact that she lived alone became the issue.

I got a call at one o'clock in the morning from my mother to tell me that her dog had gotten out and she couldn't find her anywhere.

"You went outside, Mom?" It was the dead of winter in upstate New York. No person, no dog should be outside.

"Yes, and I can't find her."

I sped the ten-minute ride to her house, all the while envisioning that her little dog was frozen somewhere on her large property or had gotten run over on her busy street. I was as frantic as my mother sounded by the time I got there. I went into her house, where she met me with tears rolling down her cold cheeks.

"Where is my dog? What happened to my dog?"

"Don't worry. I'll find her. When did you last see her? Did you look upstairs?" I looked past her down the front hall, and there was the dog—calm, cool, and curious. I was elated.

"Look, there she is. She was in the house this whole time."

My mother turned around and looked. "Not that fat dog—my *other* dog."

I just stared at her. Very calmly I said, "Mom, that's the only dog you have."

"Why do you say that? Find my poor dog."

And so it began. After days of arguing about her missing dog, out of sheer frustration I told her that her other dog was at the vet's. That kept her off the subject for a few days. Then I got a call from the vet saying that my mother had called and insisted that they return her dog. They had kept it for over a year and that was long enough. I had no choice. I killed the dog. I told her that the dog was very sick and that the vet had put her down. We mourned for days. I was feeling so depressed about the poor dead dog that didn't even exist.

I showed up for my daily visit on another winter day to find her outside, locked out in freezing weather, wearing only a skimpy red sweater. She had waited God-only-knows-how-long for me to come. She had gone looking for her beautiful cat. She doesn't have a cat. The locks were changed so that she could never lock herself out again.

Once I found a cooking pot sitting in the back hall outside her kitchen. I tried to lift it. It was burned into the carpet. There was something very charred inside the pot. When asked about it, she had no idea how it had happened. It must have been her neighbor.

Okay. That's when I began to think that things were getting dangerous. My sister and I consulted. She was even more frustrated than I, since she lived five hours away and there was nothing she could do to help the situation. Mom couldn't drive, cook, walk her dog, or go upstairs to her bedroom without risk of injury or worse. She didn't change her clothes and developed a firm dislike of washing herself. She didn't recognize her home of thirty-five years as being her own. It was agreed that Mom shouldn't be left alone and that I couldn't do it all. We got some daytime help—someone to keep her company, to cook, and to drive her around.

It was about at that time, when we were coming to terms with her situation, that the hallucinations started. There were good delusions, and there were bad delusions. The nuns living upstairs—good. The men in the woods killing animals—bad. Unfortunately, the bad greatly outnumbered the good. She would call me terrified and crying about the slaughtered animals outside and the hooligans camped in her woods. Once she called me in the middle of the night because there was a bat in her room. Naturally, I didn't believe her, but she insisted that she would call the police if I couldn't come. So I went. There was a bat in her room.

It was getting hard to separate her reality from the truth. Around three or four o'clock every afternoon, she became anxious and her hallucinations terrified her. We now had a new appreciation for the term "sundowning." I started to lie.

"Mom, I called the police, and they are going to chase them away."

"Mom, the police rounded up the hooligans, and they are all in jail."

"Mom, your other cat is sleeping upstairs."

"Yes, I saw your mother, and she is very happy."

I couldn't be speeding through town every night from her house to mine, so I started spending nights with her. I also started to sort my way through medications that were to help her with her anxieties and hallucinations but would only serve to knock her out until two o'clock the next day. Actually, sometimes that wasn't so bad.

Somehow, I managed to cope with it all until the first time she didn't know who I was. That broke my heart. Now she talks to me about me and I find it freakishly funny.

Of course, most of it wasn't one bit funny. She was up a lot during the night to look for a missing animal or to peek out the window at the bad people camped outside. I was starting to get cranky from lack of sleep. My cats weren't pleased either, because I wasn't home to give them their breakfast as soon as they woke up. My life was getting unmanageable, and something had to be done. My sister and I discussed our options and came up with a plan.

Mom is moving in with me. One day soon I will put her in the car to come visit me for a few days, and she will never see her home again. I don't know how this will work out. I will take it one day at a time and not worry about the future. It will be what it will be. I've learned that patience and a sense of humor will take me a long way. Both have been seriously tested. My mother, being a mighty opinionated French lady, has "no" as her favorite word. Translation not needed. Do you want to take a shower? No. Do you want some breakfast? No. Do you want to see the newspaper? No. Even if she really means yes, no comes out first. Now I just do, and don't ask. So I won't ask, "Mom, do you want to come and live with me?" I'll just do it. I understand that it won't be easy—for her or for me. However, this is the best decision for us at this time.

There is just one small problem: I have to tell my cats that my hallucinating mother, a real dog, and a variety of imaginary animals are coming to live with us.

—May Mavrogenis

One Brief Moment

I parked the car and tried to ignore the feeling in the pit of my stomach. Dread, heavy and cumbersome, weighed on my shoulders. I placed my head on the steering wheel. I was going to throw up. My forehead felt clammy and stuck to the steering wheel as I inhaled, counted to five, and then exhaled.

You can do this, I thought, as I lifted my head and looked toward the door.

Just once I would like to see a flash of recognition when I walked through the doors. Just once I would like Dad to smile and open his arms wide like he used to. Was that too much to ask?

"Here we go," I whispered as I opened the door of the assisted living facility.

Alzheimer's attacked Dad quickly, and in a few short months the man I knew went from loving me and my mother with all his heart to being a disori-ented and violent man. Placing him in the assisted-living facility had been our only choice after I saw the bruises on my mother.

"Honey, he didn't mean to," Mom had said. "He didn't recognize me."

She had become afraid of him, and I became afraid for them both.

On this visit, I located Dad wandering the halls, looking for Lucy, our blonde cocker spaniel that had died when I was thirteen. Searching for Lucy keeps Dad mobile and decreases his risk of bedsores. I worry that he might fall or, worse, that he might not recognize his surroundings and become violent toward the staff; but the nurses report that Dad is fine, that I shouldn't worry. I have to trust they know what is best.

As usual, I brought a basket of treats. This time I also brought an old photo album, hoping to free a memory from the grip of Alzheimer's.

"Benjamin, come over here and sit down. Look who has come for a visit," Mom said.

Dad ignored her and called again for Lucy.

"Benjamin!" she repeated and stood to get him.

Patty, the nurse who had the ability to coerce Dad to do anything, took him by the arm and steered him toward us. Dad sat down and glanced toward the basket of goodies.

"The staff here is marvelous," my mother whispered as she reached for the coffee I'd brought her. A weekly treat from Starbucks, it was the least I could do for her, especially now that she spent most of her time here.

"I don't know what I would do without them," she said, sipping her coffee.

A shiver traveled down my spine, and I prayed we never had to find out. Money had been tight since we'd moved Dad into his new home. Mom had put the house on the market, and we both hoped she would get enough from the sale of the house to pay for the care Dad needed.

"It is a tragedy to outlive your money," Mom said.

My stomach lurched again. I made a mental note to discuss with my mother where she planned to live once she sold the house. It had come down to this: My penny-pinching parents, who had saved for years so they could live comfortably after retirement, had been enjoying their golden years until a random day last year when Dad got lost on his way to the grocery store. That was the day our lives changed forever.

"Here you go, Benjamin," Patty said as she helped Dad to a seat. "You have a nice visit with your daughter."

Dad stared at me with dead eyes, and my heart sank. He didn't recognize me. He never does.

Mother placed her bony hand on my knee and pressed lightly.

"Benjamin, Renea brought you some coffee," she said as she extended the cup to him.

I miss my dad. I miss the fun we used to have, the laughter we shared, and the comfort I felt knowing that he loved me.

Dad reached into the basket and pulled out a large chocolate bar with almonds, his favorite. He unwrapped the candy and crammed most of it in his mouth.

"Have you seen Lucy?" he asked, while spewing pieces of chocolate mixed with saliva on the table.

My answer was always the same. "Dad, she's asleep at the foot of your bed."

My dad was gone. Even though I sat across the table from his body, the dad who'd raised me would never have exhibited such table manners. It was just another part of my dad that Alzheimer's had taken. Part of me wanted to wipe his mouth, another wanted to curl up in his lap like I used to and wait for him to tell me this was a bad dream.

Alzheimer's was much worse than a bad dream. For me, it was a nightmare.

Dad nodded and took a sip of coffee. "Lucy was a good girl." Coffee dribbled down his chin.

Mom reached toward Dad with a napkin to absorb the dribble, and I watched his eyes darken.

He pressed his lips tight and turned toward me as if angry to see me sitting at the table.

"Dad, it's me." I said.

Dad looked back to Mom, who nodded as if her nodding would help him remember.

Dad reached for another candy bar and said nothing. I tried not to cry. Dad can't help that he has forgotten all of us—all of us except Lucy.

Dad stared past Mom and me toward the nurse's station.

"Have you seen Lucy?" he asked another resident who was passing by. His eyes scanned the room, wild with concern.

I reach out and touched his hand. "Yes, Dad. Lucy is on your bed, asleep."

"She's a good girl." He took another sip of coffee.

I turned the page of the photo album while Dad watched the television bolted to the wall.

"Maybe the pictures weren't a good idea," Mom whispered.

"Patty said something might click," I replied.

But as I turned the crinkled pages of the tired photo album, nothing clicked.

Suddenly, Dad's attention focused on a small black-and-white photo of the three of us fishing when I was a child. He froze for a moment and looked at the picture. His fingers tapped it as if he were trying to process the photograph. Mother and I held our breath. Maybe he would remember. Maybe today would be the day.

"Would you look at this," Dad said, and a small glimmer of recollection flashed across his face.

He picked up the album and brought the picture closer. I pressed my fingers to my lips and closed my eyes. It was working; he was remembering.

"That's a picture of Lucy," Dad said while tapping the picture. He pushed the album over to my mother. "Right there," he said. "Lucy is standing in the boat beside Renea."

My heart lurched. He said my name.

Mom beamed. "That's right, Benjamin. That was Father's Day many years ago. You, Renea, Lucy, and I were all at the lake."

Mother touched Dad's hand, and her voice softened. "Do you remember that day, Benjamin?"

"Renea always was such a good girl," Dad said.

Mom's face blurred in front of me as I tried not to cry.

I'm right here, Daddy, I thought. *Please recognize me.*

"She used to outfish me something fierce," Dad said and turned to me. "Didn't you, daughter?"

He remembered. I smiled and reached for him. His hand was warm and strong as he pulled me toward him. I stood, half-stumbling, eager to hug him, and in that moment, I was his baby girl again.

"I love you, Daddy," I said as I squeezed his thin body.

Behind me, my mother blew her nose.

Dad squeezed me tight, and my heavy heart filled with the love only he could give.

"Have you seen Lucy?" he asked. "I can't seem to find her anywhere."

And my dad was gone again.

—*Renea Winchester*

Forgetting, Remembering

Alzheimer's disease has taken Mama's mind on a one-way trip back in time. I make out milestones as she reaches the ages of my grandchildren in reverse. Her spelling and handwriting is so like my kindergarten grandson that it caught me by surprise. Today my fingers guide fabric under the sewing machine for a dress for Mama. Like my five-month-old granddaughter, she will be drawn to the bright red and soft touch of the flannel fabric.

I remember when she sewed for me. She always made a new dress for my birthday. She designed the prettiest one when I was ten. The forest green and dark pink plaid dress had a pink yoke with a tab holding three pink buttons going down the left side, balanced by a pink border on the skirt and a tab coming up the right side with three matching pink buttons.

Most of the dresses came from feed sack collections donated by country church members, people who shared a way of life brought on by too much work and not enough money. They were cotton farmers with a few cows or dairy farmers with a few acres of cotton. To compensate for my father's inadequate salary as their pastor, they would share garden produce, meat when they killed hogs, and feed sacks with our family. The sacks came in attractive prints, and Mama knew how to combine them with solid-color remnants to make pretty dresses. She once copied my aunt's ready-made dress with an unusual collar and a laced up weskit. Mama's feed sack reproduction was prettier than the original!

As I hem her dress, I remember Mama teaching me to sew. Hems must be mastered first. Her instructions were exact: "With your first stitch, pick up one thread in the skirt and one thread in the hemline with your needle. Pass the needle through the fold exactly half an inch. Repeat until the hem is finished. When done correctly, the hem is invisible on the inside as well as the outside."

"What difference does it make if the hem is invisible on the inside?" I asked her. "Nobody will ever know." Being so meticulous seemed like a great deal of trouble to me at nine years old.

"*You* will know," she said.

Mama knew, too. She inspected. Her sisters, expert seamstresses themselves, also knew. Mama brought out my hems for admiration when they visited. Their awe and wonder over my invisible hems rewarded my care. I learned to love the sewing fingerwork that many seamstresses find tedious.

When Mama finished teaching me to sew, I made my clothes and sewed for my three younger sisters. They didn't check their hems on the inside, but they were invisible.

Automatically picking up one thread in the soft red flannel skirt and one in the hemline and passing the needle through one-half inch of the hem, my thoughts stray to the erosion of Mama's mind. I wonder at the things she's forgotten and the things she's remembered. Mama gave up sewing unawares. It just diminished and faded away.

One Thanksgiving when she was in the early stages of this disease, her house was filled with many relatives and much talking. My sisters and I did food preparation, stopping repeatedly at Mama's request to see how well she had swept the porch again. At mealtime, Mama, who once dominated conversations, listened and made occasional comments— some relevant, some not.

In the evening, while we finished the dishes together, Mama stared at me and asked, "Now, who are you?" We were at the end of a long day. She had coped with a big celebration. She was tired. Still, how do you tell your mother who you are? She waited for an answer.

"Mama, remember? I'm Virginia Ann."

Recognition returned. She gave an embarrassed laugh. "Oh, yes," she said.

Even as I savored the relief, I knew the time was coming soon when recognition would not return. By the next spring she couldn't remember to refrigerate leftover food, and it wasn't safe for her to live alone. She moved into an extended-care facility.

Now, I sewed for her as she had once done for me. Gwyn, the sister who lived close to Mama and was her primary caregiver, accompanied me to the rest home when I had a holiday break from teaching and could make the eight-hour trip to visit. In the beginning, Mama would gaze at me, trying to figure out who I was, until I gave her the dress I'd brought. She would brighten. "You always bring me a new dress," she'd say. After she'd forgotten my name, I was content to be the "dress lady." Now, she no longer even remembers that I'm the dress lady.

Even more difficult than Mama not knowing me is her forgetting how to read. My early memories include her readings from Tennyson, Longfellow, and the Bible. Lack of understanding of the words didn't stop my love of the rhythm and sound of her voice as she read first to three and then to four daughters. We were dressed for bed, leaning back on the pillows. Breezes floated in the windows and through the open dog-trot house. Night sounds accompanied her chosen selections. Anxious to introduce me to the wonder of words and books, she taught me to read before I started to school. How can it be that Mama can't read?

I finish the dress and wrap it in shiny paper with brightly colored bows, hoping the brilliance will reach inside her Alzheimer's eyes. If eyes are the windows of the soul, the drapes have been drawn on Mama's. I long to stand and look into those windows. I want to be invited in to talk, to listen—even to argue—but she no longer has an invitation to extend.

While she's been busy forgetting, Mama has always remembered certain things. When she prays, her voice is strong. She knows the words to every hymn. When church groups come to sing with her care facility, she holds the hymnbook for the blind woman sitting next to her. Her caring habits of a pastor's wife linger still.

Perhaps some of those habits have been passed on to me, along with her lessons on hemming. Perhaps that is why I take all of a long weekend to make the long trip even when she no longer remembers who I am. But that's only part of it. In truth, I visit Mama mostly for myself—because I still know and cherish who she is.

On my next visit, Gwyn again accompanies me, so Mama will see a familiar face.

"Mama, I've brought you something," I say, placing the gift box in her lap.

She strokes the box. She can't seem to tell how to get inside.

Gwyn asks, "Mama, do you want me to help you open it?"

"Yes, please." Mama looks relieved.

Gwyn lifts the lid. Mama looks at the bright color. Her eyes light up. She smoothes the soft fabric. Her fingers travel down to the hem. She turns it over and inspects the inside. The stitches are invisible, inside and out. Mama looks up from the hem and smiles. Her nod of approval tells me she can't see the stitches. The hem has passed. For a moment there is a sliver of recognition, a hint of remembrance.

If I take the time to do the hem right, who will know?

I will know. And maybe Mama will remember.

—*Virginia McGee Butler*

Strawberries in January

"What have you been up to?" I asked my mother as I settled into the chair across from her.

"Picking strawberries again," she said. "We have lettuce, too, even more than the rabbits can eat, so we get some."

"Really?" I said, deciding not to try to reorient her.

It was January in Pennsylvania and obviously not a day of clarity for my mother. Dementia had stolen much of her memory, and many days she was confused. She often had angry outbursts and felt left out because "nobody tells me anything." I could only imagine how frustrated and frightened she must feel. Today, however, we talked pleasantly of strawberry picking, gardening, and chicken farming—even though she didn't recognize me.

For the past several years, if she remembered me at all, it was as a small child. Often she had no memory of her two youngest children, only the older three. At first, it hurt deeply that she did not know me. Over time I came to better understand the disease, which eased the pain but not the longing for some spark of recognition.

"Mom, do you remember how you made strawberry sponge pie for my birthday? I'd request it and you made it almost every year, even after you'd taught me how to make it myself."

She just looked at me, her brow furrowed, and then hung her head.

I knew bringing up the pie and calling her Mom was a mistake. She didn't remember me or the pie, and now her light mood had shifted. At least she had been happy in her confusion this time, and now I had ruined that.

Trying to change the subject, I said, "I like that picture," as I pointed to a framed calendar photo of a fluffy, snow white kitten with a ball of yarn.

Mom's face lit up. She had already forgotten the question and was living in the moment. With a little prodding, she began talking about cats, dogs, and birds.

I excused myself to prepare a meal with the groceries I'd brought. My father had become the cook who didn't like his own cooking. Mom had forgotten how to cook, a sad realty that had become evident more than a year ago by setting the salad on fire on the stove top. I quickly prepared a simple meal of soup and salad, and when Mom wanted to help, I invited her to set the table. Having done that, she bid me good-bye.

"Time to go home," she said. "I've got to take care of the chickens and fix supper."

"Why don't you stay and have supper with us? I'm sure your family will understand," I ventured, again deciding not to reorient her.

"Oh no, I couldn't. The work never ends, you know; all I do is work."

"Well, you have to wait for your husband, anyway; he dropped you off on his way to the post office," I lied. "You might as well sit and have supper until he comes." I prayed she would accept this excuse. "Besides, I need help eating this soup. I made too much. I know you wouldn't want to waste it."

"It does smell good. I guess I could sit down and have some until he comes. That man will be late for his funeral! I suppose the work will wait a little while . . . until he comes to get me," she grumbled.

Satisfied, at least for the moment, Mom pulled out a chair and sat waiting expectantly. "Is it ready? You know I have to go."

"Coming right up, ma'am," I joked, trying to stall to give Dad time to arrive.

Dad joined us before we'd started eating, and we had a pleasant meal. Tonight, she did remember him, and she lectured him about being late and "keeping this nice lady waiting supper."

As I cleaned up the kitchen, Dad persuaded Mom to rest a bit in the easy chair. She wanted to go home. Preparing to leave, I wondered what Mom would say. She held my hands and said, "Thanks for coming; you come again when you can stay longer." In her easy chair, she was again at home.

As I drove away, I realized it had been the presence of a friendly stranger in her kitchen—me—that had confused my mother, making it seem as though she were visiting me in my home rather than the other way around. Growing up, the kitchen had been where Mom and I had shared the joys of baking, cooking, and creating. It was the one place where I felt I had my mother's attention. Hot tears filled my eyes and spilled over my cold cheeks. Dementia continued to steal from us, and I was helpless to stop it.

The following April, Dad had a pacemaker implanted, and then six months later he suffered a stroke. At eighty-eight years of age and incapacitated by illness, he made it very clear there were to be no hospitals for him. He was ready to die, and he wanted to die at home.

Mom couldn't comprehend his failing health even in those fleeting moments when she knew him.

Another stroke rendered Dad bedridden and unresponsive. Once or twice, Mom asked where he'd gone, looking out the window toward the fields.

I prayed. I tried to prepare Mom for Dad's death, carefully explaining to her that he was very ill and taking her to his room. She looked and left—clearly not connecting the man in the bed with the man with whom she'd lived for nearly seventy years. Hospice came to help. Dad died a few days later, going home to be with Jesus, his heart's desire.

I worried how Mom would react if she saw Dad's body removed. It was agreed I would distract her with an old photo album she enjoyed. She never noticed the activity around her. She seemed engrossed in times long past.

The next day we moved Mom to a loving personal-care home, where she had resided for a time several years before. She seemed pleased by the warm reception and a task to do, peeling potatoes. I was relieved that she seemed so happy and content, yet I was disturbed that she didn't miss Dad. He'd been her one connection to the present and to reality for years.

Concerned about how she would react, I took Mom to Dad's funeral an hour before people were to arrive. Along the way, I pointed out things I hoped she would find familiar and then told her where we were going. Many funerals of family and friends had been held there. She didn't remember.

As I guided her to the casket, she remarked about all the chairs several times. We stood at the casket. I held my breath. She looked, expressionless and then puzzled. "Well, I don't know him. Why did you bring me here? Let's go. I have work to do." She turned and mused again, "They sure have a lot of chairs."

I drove her back to the home while fighting back tears. Mom couldn't understand. It seemed so cruel. The pain in my chest grew. I prayed and then glanced over at Mom. She was enjoying the sunny day and the blue skies. When she saw a bird fly so close it almost touched the glass, she smiled. She wasn't grieving.

Then, like the brilliance of the light streaking the skies at sunrise, it dawned on me: Dementia had robbed her of a great deal, but it had also taken her grief. She did not recall the pain of burying two daughters. In her mind, if she remembered them at all, they were happy, healthy, boisterous children. She did not feel like she'd been cut in half by the loss of her husband. If she remembered him, it would be to wonder why he stayed so long in the fields. She no longer remembered the scars and shame of her illegitimate birth and the abuse of her childhood and youth. The memory loss that had caused so much pain, anger, and frustration for her in the beginning of the disease now proved to be a friend, erasing and eliminating her heartache.

For the remainder of her life, Mom lived content and happy, oblivious to the stresses of daily life, unburdened by sorrows and regrets. She enjoyed walking under falling snowflakes in July and picking strawberries in January.

There is little to commend dementia. It is devastating to everyone touched by it. But in that moment, I recognized that even in the worst of times, God provides a ray of hope and a blessing, if only we can recognize them.

—*Jeanne Wilhelm*

Lest We Forget, Thank You

My sister, Donna, called me, frantic. "Erika, we have to do something about Dad."

Of course we did. My father's accountant had phoned me shortly before April 15: Dad could not locate needed documents. His lifelong friend's wife had phoned concerned: Dad got lost en route to the house they'd lived in for fifty years. My dad's "woman friend," too, had recounted her worries over the telephone: Dad could not travel alone to visit my brother in Puerto Rico; she must go with him, or he would forget his wallet.

I live in North Carolina. At the time, Dad lived in New Jersey, where he had been born eighty-six years earlier.

"Dad wants to go to his high school reunion, which is being held in West Orange," said Donna in

Chicago. "You know he'll get lost if he tries to drive there. Can you fly up and take him?"

The youngest of my four children had just finished her junior year of high school. Two sons were enrolled in summer semesters at their colleges; the other was busily working. I had the time available. My husband said, "Go."

I arranged to be picked up by the same limousine driver who often transported my dad to and from the airport when he went on his many overseas vacations. When we reached Dad's house, Sam knocked on the front door as he held my luggage. I rang the bell. No answer. It was 1:30 PM, and I had spoken with Dad the night before. Where could he be?

I went around to the back door and knocked. No answer. So I peered through the windows into the once tidy den, which was now cluttered with piles of newspapers, letters, books, and junk mail. The door leading from the den to the attached greenhouse was swung open, and inside I could see overturned pots and weeds growing in containers that had once held spouts. When I turned around, I saw that the back yard was in no better shape. Though it was mid-summer, the pool cover had not been taken off, and puddles of algae muck had settled in the creases. The lawn looked as if Dad were growing hay. The once well-kept vegetable garden had not even been planted.

It suddenly dawned on me that things had changed for my father more radically than I had assumed.

I went back around to the front of the house and hollered outside his bedroom window. "Dad! Dad! Are you there?"

"Do you have a key to the house?" asked Sam.

"No."

"Is there one hidden?"

"Not that I know of."

I could see in Sam's eyes that he thought me woefully inadequate for the job ahead.

As Sam was shaking his head, the window creaked open above us in my parents' bedroom. Out popped an old white head with a big smile and a shirtless torso. "Hi, Erika! What are you doing here?" Dad called out cheerfully.

It was as though I lived down the street and had popped in unexpectedly at an early hour. In reality, I have lived away from home since college in 1969. He did not seem aware that I had flown there from North Carolina just to take him to his high school reunion the next day. He seemed to have no concept of time.

I spent that next week with Dad, cleaning his house, paying overdue bills, taking him out to eat, visiting with his friends, contracting with lawn and pool people to clean up his acre lot, and of course, going to his reunion—the Weequahic High School of Newark, New Jersey's Class of 1937.

Dad said he knew the way. Why I did not tuck a map into his car is my failing, but at that point in time, I think I had not really accepted the fact that my dad had Alzheimer's. He seemed to think I knew the way, as if I were my mother who had been born in West Orange and is now buried there. He often said on the trip, "Well, Shirley—I mean, Erika—you know where this place is. You've been there before." I had not. I'm sure my mother had.

He became very agitated with me when we got lost in the "down neck" section of Newark. It was a hot June day, and although we had left early enough to get to the reunion on time, we were already a half hour late. I asked a gas attendant who spoke broken English for directions; he drew me a map.

Dad had lost faith and was stewing. He told me to forget it and just go home. "I don't want to go now," he said. "We missed it."

I drove on with a sullen passenger. When we arrived at the Italian restaurant, everyone was eating dessert. However, the staff, all of whom were Italian, was very accommodating and fetched the salad and chicken dish prepared for us.

Each of the nineteen invitees stood and recounted what they were doing now, how many grandchildren they had, and how blessed they were with whatever arrangement they had. I was the only child of a graduate there, and some mistook me for a much younger second wife. (At that point, I, too, felt like it was a mistake being there.)

When it was Dad's turn, he stood up. "Well, I don't do much. I sleep a lot." Then, he paused, about to sit down, and one woman asked him how many grandchildren he had. "Ah, let me think. ... Erika, how many do I have?"

"Seven, Dad."

"That's right. Seven."

Another woman asked what he had done for a living before he retired.

"I got fired."

I think Dad meant it as joke. No one asked him any more questions. I murmured to Dad that he should tell them how glad he was to see them all again.

"Manny," he turned to the class president, "Remember when we set off that pipe bomb in the bathroom?"

Manny chuckled.

"And remember . . . oh, what was that history teacher's name who told that Italian kid to be on time and the kid said he couldn't because he always had to take a bowel movement before class, and then Mr. So and So told him to regulate his bowel movements better?" Dad laughed.

Everyone else was silent, except Dad's old friend Manny, who chuckled a bit. Me, I had my napkin almost covering my face. But I peaked out, and Dad looked happy. He sat down, still grinning.

I was sort of glad things wound down quickly after Dad's speech. A few wanted the class to pose for pictures, and I couldn't have been happier to be the photographer and not the photographed. Dad was in the midst of all the shots, smiling. He wandered about, talking with different couples, and then everyone seemed to exit simultaneously. Most called cabs.

When Dad and I got into the car to head home, he turned to me. "Erika, before I forget to tell you, thank you. Thank you so much for taking me."

"It's okay, Dad. It really was nothing. I was glad to do it for you."

"No, it was a lot of trouble. And I want you to know that I appreciate it. I might forget to tell you later. You may not have noticed, but I forget a lot of stuff."

I glanced over at my dad to see if he were making a joke. He wasn't.

"You are a good daughter."

We drove back to his house. When I left New Jersey at the end of the week, I took Dad with me to North Carolina. Several other trips back to Jersey were made to sell the house. Now Dad lives with me and my husband in our empty nest.

This year, Manny called to say there would be a seventieth high school reunion at a restaurant in West Orange. With a little creative planning and the help of Sam's limo service, my dad attended— without me. He told me he had a swell time. I asked him what they talked about.

"You know, Erika, my memory is not so good. I really don't know. But I know I had a good time. Thank you, Honey."

That's what it all boils down to: "I had a good time. ... Thank you, honey."

Do I wish Dad could converse more coherently and remember what I served him for breakfast each day? Of course! But when I see his eyes glow with happiness and when he looks at me and says "thank you," it is enough. I, too, am thankful—that I am still someone's child and that I can pay back my dad for all he's done for me.

—*Erika Hoffman*

The Triumph of Love

I have seen her.

You may think that's wishful thinking on my part. If you're looking for evidence, you've got the wrong gal. I don't have to convince you of anything … and I know what I saw.

I'd been walking through my living room one December evening and stopped to gaze at my Christmas tree glittering before the front window with hundreds of tiny white lights. It was one of those pre-lit jobs that are so bright that, when I plugged it in, the entire Shenandoah Valley went dark.

Just kidding.

The tree itself was an issue for me. My first "fake" tree. I felt like a traitor. My kids were not pleased with me, but my kids had moved out and moved on. I fully accept that a "real" Christmas tree is nostalgic as heck, but taking the blasted thing down every year had become more than I could handle. It's not that I'm old and weak. It's just that I'm lazy. I wasn't worried about the kids. Being my children all their lives, they had learned how to adjust to all levels of strangeness. I knew that, in time, they'd come to embrace the synthetic tree, especially since it would have genuine presents under it when they showed up on Christmas Eve.

The guilt that ate at me that night had nothing to do with the kids. It had to do with her. She'd always been the source of Christmas joy and richness and magic and beauty for me. Under her tutelage, I learned about Father Christmas long before Santa Claus held any importance in my life. Because of her, I know the taste of plum pudding and hard sauce. Because of her, I can make an acceptable trifle. Because of her, I am well-versed in the details and intricacies of serving both an afternoon tea and a formal high tea. Because of her, I love shortbread, and because of her, no matter who sings "Silent Night," all my heart hears is the warm, lovely sound of England.

That woman could sing, let me tell you.

Britannia passed gracefully through her every time she spoke and every time she sang. The country of kings and uprisings, of Shakespeare and Marlowe, of

J. K. Rowling and Dickens. The country of Elizabeth the First, Victoria, Jack the Ripper, Sherlock Holmes, and Tony Blair. The country of Celts and Saxons and The Knights of the Round Table. This was her homeland, and I lived in awe of its mark upon her.

I can say with total confidence that I was her favorite grandchild. I know this because, every time I asked her (which was often), she'd shake her head, chuckle, and say, "Aren't you dreadful for asking me such a thing?"

I'd reply with, "Please note, you did not tell me no. Therefore, the answer is yes."

Then she'd walk away, still shaking her head and still chuckling, and murmur back at me, "Aren't you naughty?"

My predictable reply, "I am. You love it, baby."

And she'd start laughing all over again.

As much as she was utterly English, I am utterly American. We utterly clashed often. Generally, my vulgar, tomboyish comportment seemed to be the issue. Who knew simple whistling could cause so much trouble? Well, I knew—since she made it her quest to correct me every time I started—therefore, I whistled constantly.

Her reaction: "Must you be so vulgar?"

My response: "Whistling is not vulgar. Whistling topless would be vulgar."

Her return volley: "Oh, how dreadful!"

And on and on and on.

Of course, she loved me best. That should be obvious.

I loved her—and still love her—insanely, so when those piercing blue eyes of hers started to go blank, I retreated immediately into denial. The whole world might go barking mad, but she never would. Not my grandmother. No. She was too proper, too formal, too decent, too honorable, too generous, too pious, too good to be crushed by the ugly, heartless predator of Alzheimer's.

No. That's all I could say, and it's all I still say. No.

I watched her slip into darkness, and my chest convulsed with hatred for a God who would allow it. Let the rest of us get what we've got coming to us. That should satisfy any eternal accountant and balance the books. But she did nothing, nothing, nothing to deserve such a thing. My grandmother taught me to pray. She taught the entire family to pray. That the God she trusted and believed in so unwaveringly should sit silently by and watch her mind be devoured by Alzheimer's caused me the most intense period of religious doubt I have ever known. I will not survive another one like it.

I'm not sure I survived even that one. Eleven years have gone since she was taken away from me and still, I sit here and weep because I miss her so.

The time came when she no longer recognized me. I'd see her sitting in a chair with her lifeless eyes staring at nothing. I'd sit beside her, take her hand in mine, and say, "Hey, Grandma."

Those eyes would blink, turn toward me, but never focus.

I did not cry at her funeral. I would like to have cried, but there was nothing inside me, save the constant blowing of a cold wind. Over and over, my mind grappled with the mystery of how my grandmother could be reduced to a grammatical lesson in verb conjugation.

She is.

She was.

Gone. Just gone.

Days and weeks went by. I felt nothing. The old gal was dead. I understood. No problem. Life sucks, but that's the way it goes. Time to buck up.

Weeks became months. Then Christmas. Something inside me twinged. I took a deep breath, fought it, and made it through Christmas.

She'd been gone a year and a half, and my life was back to normal. Everyone loses a grandparent sooner or later. Are we all supposed to just hit the brakes and drop in our tracks? I think not. We go on. Period. So that's what I did.

Then one day at the grocery store, I rounded a corner from one aisle to another, and there she was, peering at something or other on one of the shelves. I stopped so hard, the contents of my cart shifted forward with a loud clatter. I knew that brown-grey hair, that long, aristocratic nose, the pretty blue dress (to match her eyes), and even those glasses. I could recognize them all, blindfolded. I could not breathe. My mind rebelled, but my heart shouted to her. Cold logic wrestled savagely with jubilation so overwhelming I feared my knees would buckle.

She turned to look at me and, instantly, I realized my mistake. Very close, but not her. She watched me inquiringly, her brilliant blue eyes making my chest heave, and she asked softly, "Are you all right, my dear?"

Those soft English syllables. My head began to spin.

I nodded, tried to smile, and managed, "Please forgive me for staring. I thought you were . . . see, . . . the thing is, . . . I thought you were . . . well, I apologize."

She stepped toward me, put a hand against my arm, and asked, "Has she been gone a long time, my dear?"

I tried to speak, but the words garbled in my throat. I looked away and breathed, "Not long. About eighteen months. I don't think I can stand it much more. I thought I was okay, but I'm not. I can't bear it. I can't."

She reached up and put her arms around me, and the pain I had jammed down for so long surged forward in mighty waves. I sobbed against the woman's shoulder for a long time. She spoke soothingly to me. In my heart, I heard, *There, there, my darling. There, there. What's wrong with Grandma's little treasure girl? There, there. We must be brave, mustn't we?*

I can't say how long I stood there in the grocery store weeping in this gentle old woman's arms. Maybe a few minutes. Maybe longer. When I finally stopped and stepped back, the stranger smiled up at me and asked, "Feeling a little better, perhaps?"

I smiled, shrugged, and said yes.

She smiled back and said, "She's never far away. You'll remember that, won't you?"

"Yes, ma'am. I'll remember."

Such emotional outbursts always embarrass me, so I turned my cart around and walked away faster than courtesy would dictate. Then I felt ashamed of myself for leaving her so quickly, so I turned around and stepped back into the aisle. She was gone.

Years later, on a winter's night, I stood in front of my first "fake" Christmas tree and tried to imagine what my grandmother might say. I worried and fretted and considered whether I should take it down and get a "real" one.

Behind me, in the silence, I heard a familiar voice, "What nonsense."

I smiled. In the window's reflection, I could see her standing behind me, her purse clutched in her hands. She leaned forward, eyeing my Christmas tree with a critical expression I knew all too well.

"You think it's okay?" I whispered, watching her in the reflection.

"Of course I do. It's perfectly lovely."

"It's fake," I admitted uneasily.

"No matter. It's a lovely tree."

"I thought you wouldn't like it."

"What nonsense," she said again.

"I miss you."

"Don't be such a silly child. I'm never far away."

"I love you, Grandma."

"Tut-tut," she replied impatiently.

I grinned, and I know I saw her smile back at me. Then, she faded away.

But she will never fade away. Even the powerful, heartless Alzheimer's could not rob me of her. I remember her smile. I remember the sound of her voice and the fullness of her laughter. Alzheimer's took what it could get, and all it could get was her mind. Her soul and her spirit escaped and live on. The images and nightmare of her death (which took eight years) have faded enough that other memories have taken their rightful place inside me.

Shall I tell the horrific details of her descent into the black pit of the disease? Shall I recount the end-less humiliations her person endured? Shall I explain what happens to an elegant, intelligent, compassion-ate, loving human being when her keen mind is leeched away from her without warning?

Well, I won't. Anyone who has ever watched a loved one destroyed by the scourge of Alzheimer's already knows those hideous details.

This was my grandmother. I loved her—and still love her—insanely, and Alzheimer's did not win. Alzheimer's lost, because she is still close to me.

Will I ever recover from her death? No. But everything wonderful about her lives on inside me and inside my children and, someday, inside my grandchildren.

She taught me a love for words. She taught me, by example, how a dignified woman presents herself. She taught me that being honest is more important than being right. She taught me to trust God, even when I didn't think He deserved it.

Alzheimer's does not win. Not ever. Love wins, and the triumph of love over death is eternal.

—Camille Moffat

A Timeless Gift

A great cloud of dust arose as I lifted the large canvas tarp that concealed my attic treasure. My heart pounded with excitement as the dust settled to reveal the masterpiece, the monument of memories—the Great Temple of Tongue Depressors!

My thoughts drifted back thirty years to one magical Christmas. I was only seven then, but there are some memories a child never forgets . . . the same kind of special memories you hope your parents will never forget. As I ran my finger across the dirty surface of my precious gift, I recalled every detail of that year. My patience had been challenged and my curiosity had been insatiable all the months I kept vigil outside my father's workshop, wondering what he was creating. With an eye glued to the keyhole, I could discover only one clue: tongue depressors, lots and lots of tongue depressors.

Christmas morning finally arrived. A green bed sheet and a beautiful red bow hid the contents of the gift Daddy had made for me. I held my breath as if I were preparing to blow out birthday candles. My dad grinned from ear to ear as he cast aside the sheet, revealing the dream of all girlish dreams, the most extraordinary Victorian dollhouse I had ever seen. It was painted a classic French blue with white trim around the doors, windows, and delicate railings surrounding the decks. The two-story mansion stood nearly level with my height, was fully furnished and wallpapered and had stairs leading to the upper floor and attic.

Now, as I ran my hand over the roof the sharp iron weather vane pricked my finger. I flicked it and watched it spin, and as I did so, my thoughts returned to my father. I wanted to embrace him like I did when I was seven. I wanted to thank him all over again, even if he couldn't remember why. That was the torturing question: could he remember?

I decided to call him. I had to. After several rings, I was about to hang up when a familiar, but aged, voice answered.

"Hi, Dad!"

"Oh, hi, Julie!" he replied.

"Nope, it's your other daughter. I just wanted to call and say hi."

"Sorry it took me so long to get to the phone. I was sorting slides on the computer. I'll be finishing the China trip soon. I'll send you a DVD when I'm done."

I was thrilled to hear that he was doing something mentally stimulating to keep him from becoming too depressed about his flagging memory. I hoped the photos would prompt some of the memories of our past travels.

"Hey, Dad, guess what I was just looking at?"

"What?" The lack of enthusiasm in his tone suggested that he was anxious to get back to his project.

"Remember that dollhouse you built me?"

A long pause. I knew he was trying to remember.

"Where in the world did you get all those tongue depressors, anyway?" I asked.

"Oh, that!"

I was relieved that he could recollect some of the details that made up one of my favorite memories ever.

"A doctor friend ordered them for me. I remember that was quite a project. It took me months to get that thing built. I enjoyed it, though."

"Well, I think I might need to invest in some more of those big Popsicle sticks. Looks like some of the siding is coming loose. Luckily, the roof is still intact. How long did it take you to cut all those end pieces for the shingles?"

"Oh, I don't remember." The words were becoming a familiar reply.

"Well, maybe during your next visit you can help me fix it up. I know it will be a few years before Haley can play with it, but I know she'll love it just as much as I did."

"Yeah, I suppose we can do that. I don't think there's any hurry, though."

I silently disagreed. The last time I had seen him he was worried he wouldn't be able to watch his only granddaughter grow up. Now I was worried he would forget her. I spent the next few moments bragging about her toddler achievements before he suddenly interjected and mentioned he was making a DVD of our China trip. Looking for the brighter side of his dementia, I was pleased to hear him sound just as excited as the first time he'd told me about his project.

We hung up, and a few minutes later my sister called.

"Hey, Mitz. I wanted to talk to you about Dad. I went to his house yesterday. I'm not sure I should tell you, because he wants to tell you in person when he comes to see you in a couple weeks, but I thought we should talk about it first."

"Tell me," my voice quivered. I was frightened that she was about to reveal something disastrous, like he had been diagnosed with cancer or something. I still grieved for my mother, who had lost that battle years ago.

There was a sniffle on the other line before she spoke. "Dad was diagnosed with Alzheimer's disease."

A long pause passed before I could answer. "I hate being eight hundred miles away from you guys!" I cried. I was trying to mask the dark thoughts that penetrated my mind. I was sad but not terribly surprised. We had suspected as much for some time now.

"He's getting worse," said Julie. "A few days ago he was pulling out of the parking lot in his van when some people walked out behind him. He couldn't remember where the brakes were, and his feet kept hitting the floorboard. Pedestrians kept yelling at him to stop. Fortunately, nobody was hurt."

A cold sensation swept through my chest. I began to choke on my tears. "Is he going to lose his license? That would devastate him. He's only sixty-three. He's too young!"

"I don't know yet," she answered. "He's still in the early stages of the disease. I think he just had a bad episode."

I knew those episodes. Just a few months before, while visiting my brother in Washington, Dad suddenly became horribly confused and couldn't count his change. Since then, his struggle with short-term memory loss had increased. We all knew that within a few years he might not know us at all.

After a good sisterly cry, Julie and I hung up.

I went back up to the attic and began studying every detail of the dollhouse. From the hand-carved curves on the side molding to the tiny brass doorknob, I absorbed every ounce of workmanship that went into that creation. My father was a brilliant man. As an architect, he had crafted homes, museums, and other buildings that were every bit as nice. I was privileged to have spent my childhood in some of the homes that he had designed and built.

At that moment I realized that my dad was more than a father to me. He was my inspiration. Whenever he made up his mind to do something, he just did it, no doubts and no worries. Sorrow sagged against my heart as I became aware of his diminishing talents.

To distract my thoughts, I licked my finger in hopes of resealing some of the peeling wallpaper in the dollhouse, but my lips began to tremble and my eyes grew sore from fighting tears. Finally, I gave in and let them fall as fears flooded my mind and thoughts of becoming a virtual orphan overcame me. I was afraid of losing even a part of him and afraid I would vanish from his mind before he ultimately lost his battle with Alzheimer's.

A few days later the family had a conference call to discuss treatments, holistic remedies, long-term care, and how to cope with Dad's disease. My dad's new wife was in no hurry to put him in a home, but we made sure she would not be burdened with the weight of his illness.

Later, when my dad came to visit me in Arizona, his subtle criticism and invariable forgetfulness were repeated throughout the day. Sometimes he couldn't even remember if he had eaten his breakfast. It tested my patience, but I had prepared myself with creative ways of explaining things to him.

My father was not one to sit still for a visit, so I busied him with small projects. It made him feel important to keep active, but even the smallest things that he had once handled with ease became a source of frustration for him.

"I can't think as clearly as I used to," he admitted. "It takes me four times as long to get things done."

"Hanging screen doors and building dog houses aren't exactly things I could easily figure out," I said.

Instead of providing me with reassurance, he became more irritated.

"I can't even do my job anymore. I keep making mistakes and have to check my work over and over. The calculations don't make much sense to me anymore."

It seemed pointless to remind him that he was retired. I urged him to talk, to tell me the secret that he had already revealed to my siblings. He wouldn't open up, and by the time his visit was nearly over, I had to prompt him to talk.

"Dad, how are you feeling these days? Is there anything you want to talk about?"

"Oh, well the diabetes seems to be under control, but I have been having some problems with my memory."

"I heard you went to see a specialist."

"Yeah, they think I have some problems with forgetfulness. But I've been talking to other friends my age, and they claim to forget things too."

So maybe Dad was in denial. Either he couldn't admit that it had anything to do with the dreaded word "Alzheimer's" or he had forgotten the diagnosis altogether.

Switching to a more comfortable topic, I suggested we have a crack at fixing up the old dollhouse.

"What dollhouse?" he asked. He patted me on the shoulder with a smile. "Don't look so sad; I was just kidding. Some things I can't forget. One of them is the look on your face when I gave you that dollhouse."

I hoped that was true. I hoped he would someday see the same joy on his granddaughter's face. It seemed doubtful now, but I wanted him to help fix it up while he still knew how.

Off came the tarp, and we assessed the damage. We laughed at how the old house had incurred its injuries over the years. I reminded him of how the family cat thought it was his playhouse and how my brother's football had landed on its deck and got stuck in the French doors. We had a good laugh as we repaired the damage to the deck railings and applied new wallpaper to the interior. We created memories that will stay with me for as long as I will remember.

"I hope I get the chance to watch Haley grow up," he smiled, a sad expression shadowing his face. "Maybe her children will get to play with this doll-house someday."

"And their children," I added.

I reminded my father that his dollhouse was more than a toy. He had produced a legacy. Even if he couldn't remember, others would remember him for it. He had created a magical gift that would be passed through the generations, building everlasting memories for each child fortunate enough to behold it on their special Christmas morning. Each would carry that joy with them throughout adulthood, along with the memory of a great man whose brilliant mind had conceived of and crafted such a timeless gift.

—*Mitzi L. Boles*

Sweets for the Journey

All things considered—it was the holidays, our mother had recently been diagnosed with Alzheimer's, and the entire family was stuffed into Mom's tiny two-bedroom home—we were having as much fun as could be expected on this Christmas day. I sought refuge in the kitchen. The smell of garlic wafted from the old-fashioned electric cooker. The gourmet sausages we had brought with us sizzled nicely. In the living room, Belgian chocolates sat on the mantle. Food was always a safe option for me, the returning prodigal. It was the one thing I could provide that Mom wouldn't be disappointed in.

She looked good; she hadn't changed much since the last time I'd seen her. The familiar twinge of guilt at moving away hardly registered on my radar these days. Time flew by, and life was busy: husband, teenage son, deadlines for articles. The journey to my mother's home wasn't overly long, but there never seemed to be quite enough time for it.

I heard shuffling behind me and turned, surprised to see my mother lowering herself onto a kitchen chair in front of a bowl of carrots.

"Do you want them in rounds or slices?" she asked.

"Doesn't matter, Mom—any way you like."

She smiled and set to work, quietly focused on the carrots. I continued cooking, unable to figure out what was out of place. *Was it her smile, or was it that she seemed out of place in the kitchen, a place I rarely saw her in?*

"Do you want them in rounds or slices?"

"I already said, Mom, it doesn't matter—any way you like."

After lunch, we all sat and watched television, a Christmas movie, Kate and Leo, arms outstretched to a glorious sunset.

"I saw the Titanic, you know?" Mom said.

Philip, adored grandson since birth (was it churlish of me to be so jealous?), looked up from where he lounged on the carpet at her feet.

"No, Vic, you can't have," my aunt's voice was terse. Her face flashed with the briefest spasm of exasperation. She busied herself with the china tea cups.

"Yes, I have," Mom insisted. "I saw it . . . oh, I don't know where."

"When was that, Nanny?" Philip asked.

"Last year."

The cups clattered furiously. We all turned politely back to our tea and cookies.

Later, as we were leaving, Mom took hold of my hand, looked me straight in the eye, and said, "I love you."

Now, I knew something was wrong.

The call came a few months later. As in all the best dramas, a terrific storm was blowing. I arrived home windblown and over-excited from a dinner party. It was Philip who had taken the message.

"Nanny's in the hospital."

I immediately phoned my aunt. She had finally given up, she said. She was tired of hiding the truth, exhausted from sleepless nights trying to stop Mom from wandering when she wanted to go "home." She was scared of the increasingly physical outbursts, and she was resentful of the stranger who had replaced her sister.

Our conversation was sad and bitter. I had only ever been a phone call away. Why had she not listened to my advice to seek help? Why had she stubbornly refused all the support we had tried to arrange for her?

Worst of all, the more I railed at her, the more that tiny familiar nugget of blame started twisting around in my gut. Wasn't it me who had left, setting out into the far-off world, journeying to exotic places to mix with diplomats and politicians? Truth be told, the glamour was convenient, a citadel where I could hold myself removed, behind the sent photographs and the day-late birthday cards. How could I be demanding confidences now? Where, now, was my claim to intimacy?

We crossed the English Channel again on a clear day. My husband, Jesus, took his vacation early to accompany me, and we stood together on the deck surrounded by tourists. The little ferry ploughed through bright sunshine, but a light fog over the English coast seemed malicious and brooding, and the famous white chalk cliffs looked piqued and jaundiced. We had decided Philip shouldn't cancel his planned trip around Europe with friends, and suddenly looking at all the smiling families, I had the sensation of being sandwiched between two losses. I knew that things with Mom would never be the same, and now my son was halfway grown up and on his way to leaving me.

We traveled to Devon on small country roads, avoiding the highway, and by the time we arrived, it was dark. The night was balmy, the smell of cow manure rich through the car's open windows. It was good to breathe it in. I turned to Jesus, remembering and repeating to him something my mother used to say: "You'll never die with that smell in your nostrils."

The next day, on the way to see Mom, we bought grapes and chocolate from the local gas station.

Brunel Lodge was a small building on the outskirts of town. From over the wall, I glimpsed a patio and yard. The day was hot, and the doors were all flung open. We opened the main door, pressed the red security buzzer, and waited nervously. A plainclothes nurse greeted us with a hearty smile, and for a brief moment, it was a relief to see that someone seemed to think all this was normal. The code on the security lock was 1-2-2-5, she explained, Christmas day, easy to remember. I thought there was a touch of ironic cruelty to it.

Mom was sitting alone at a small table, looking ahead at nothing in particular. I approached her slowly, and she looked up. Then it happened. Her smile was weak, but something came alive in her eyes. She was my mom, and she was happy to see me. The unfamiliar surroundings suddenly weren't quite so frightening. It was the most natural thing in the world to hold on to her tight and tell her how good it was to see her.

The grapes disappeared quickly, shared between us. The chocolate bar was even better. Mom had always had a sweet tooth. When I was small, we would go to the beach, and she would buy huge vanilla ices topped with a dollop of thick Devonshire cream. Every day now, at the start of our visit, we would unload a small collection of sugar fruits, lollies, and chocolate bars.

We spent long afternoons sitting on a bench in the patio. It was hard to think of conversation. Well, there was really nothing new in that. But I learned new things. I read to her from a book of poems. She read to me two or three times over a few sentences from the blurb on the back of a novel someone had left lying around. We took slow turns around the tiny yard, me holding onto her arm, Mom explaining about the plants and flowers. I cut her fingernails. The skin on her hands was creamy pale, soft, and unblemished. Other people said that she wasn't herself any longer. Holding on to her arm, I thought she was the closest thing to "Mom" I would ever see.

Saying good-bye each evening was a lengthy process.

"I'll just get my handbag," she would say.

"No, Mom, you have to stay here."

"Well, where are you going to stay tonight? You haven't had a proper meal." Then looking around crossly, she'd say, "I'm sorry, but I'm having a few problems with the kitchen staff."

Sometimes, we just slipped away. Sometimes, she was calm and waved good-bye happily. "Drive safely. Take this for the journey." And she would press back into our hands what was left of the candy we had brought for her.

We were the eye of the storm. Outside of it, the whole world was changing. There were family squabbles about money. There was the small group of lifelong friends, who had claimed so much of her time before, that were now, curiously, too busy to visit. There were consultations with busy nurses and doctors and talk of psychotic episodes.

Soon, it would be time for me to leave again. With no psychiatrist to be found in our small Devonshire village, I found myself in desperation one evening paying a visit to mum's pastor, Monty. He lived with his family in a decidedly unchic, one-story home on the main road. Noting the paintwork could do with a bit of a touch-up, I knocked on the glass door, a little embarrassed to impose on him like this—I, a confirmed agnostic. Before long, I saw an athletic-looking form approaching rapidly. When the door opened, I was surprised to see a small, wiry, gray-haired man. The outline behind the glass had led me to expect someone much younger. I introduced myself a bit nervously.

A warm smile spread over his face. "Alison, come in," his rural accent breathed energy.

Over mugs of hot tea, we talked about my mother.

"Now is the time for forgiveness," said Monty.

"Yes," I replied politely, not really knowing to whom he was referring. *Was I to forgive my aunt for abandoning us all? Was she to forgive me for not being there? Were we all to forgive Mom for leaving us?*

"You know, whenever I visited your mom, before the tea was even poured she would be telling me all about you and what you were up to."

"Really?"

"Oh, yes," he nodded. "The photos would come out, and I'd have to hear all about it. You were a delight to her—you, your life, your family."

On the slow walk up the lane home that evening, the sun was low in the sky, and a slight chill nipped the air. Fall was chasing after summer. A thought struck me: maybe it was time for me to forgive myself.

Over the next few months, I traveled back and forth from my adopted home in Belgium to my childhood home in England. Each time, I saw that I'd lost a little more of my mother; each time I gained a little more of her to take away with me. Between visits, our nightly telephone calls were usually quirky, sometimes distressing and other times graceful, but often comforting. The winter days grew shorter, and so did our telephone conversations, as Mom could no longer hang on to sentences.

"What are you wearing?" ... "What can you see out of the window?" ... "I love you, Mom."

"And I love you," always strong and loud on the last word.

Our lives were busy. Philip had exams, and Jesus and I both had a lot of work. But with Mom's condition growing steadily worse, one rainy day in January, as I was preparing to make one of my regular trips over, a sudden instinct told me we should all go. We went by car, racing through the rain-glossed fields.

When the time came, we were all there with her: Jesus, Philip, my aunt, and me. I lay my head down on the bed beside my mother and said my final good-bye.

The next day we went to the nursing home to collect my mother's things. Philip was the one who found it—there, melted and mashed into the blue vinyl pocket of her walking frame, was her hidden stash of chocolate, saved especially for me. No matter how far from her I traveled, she was always happy to give me candy for the journey.

My mother had waited one last time for me to come home, and finally, I knew it had been okay for me to leave.

—*Alison Jane Light*

Waiting for Mary Lou

B y the time I met Ray, he was already sliding into the darkness, but not so far that others had really caught on yet. He was tall and patrician-looking, with enough presence of mind to bluff his way through difficult situations. For example, even after his son, Bill, and I had been married a couple of years, he never said my name. With a twinkle in his eye, he'd call me his "girlfriend." Even though Ray had some hearing loss, he wore a pretty good set of hearing aids, so it seemed a little odd to me. I was his son's second wife, so I never got a chance to meet the real Ray, though I hear he had been quite a humdinger.

I had never had a father of my own, so I enjoyed listening to the stories about my new father-in-law and imagining how Ray's life must have been when he was younger. According to the stories, Ray had married my mother-in-law, Mary Lou, during the Second World War while serving as an officer in the U.S. Navy. Even when I knew him, decades later, he still reveled in telling the story of how the bridal party had departed for the church in a flurry of excitement and left him and his bride's father at the house with no way to join them. I can picture him standing on the front porch in his naval officer's uniform, waiting for someone to remember him. Apparently, it all worked out, because they ended up married for more than fifty years. And over the years, he really enjoyed telling that story and embarrassing his "bride."

The story of their marriage doesn't end at the wedding, of course. After the war Ray went on to become an attorney and later a judge. He worked on many important cases, taught classes for the Navy and the University of Washington, and even had his own local television show. Because there was no hospital in his area to serve his young family, he and some friends formed a board and got a hospital built. Ultimately, the hard work paid off for his wife, who has been a patient there several times over the last few years.

Ray was a mover and a shaker almost all his life. He was the father of four and grandfather of many. He was involved in scouting for many years. After they retired, he and Mary Lou traveled the world. They loved to dance and belonged to a dance group for quite some time. They also stayed active in all sorts of social and service clubs. He was the most interesting and powerful man I have ever almost known personally. Unfortunately, I'd missed my father-in-law's heyday by a margin, and now we were watching him become someone the family didn't recognize.

Not only was it difficult to see my father-in-law's decline and the effect it had on the family, but it also made me worry about my husband and even myself. We had only recently found one another and married. Bill is kind, funny, thoughtful, and devoted—everything I had always wanted in a companion. What if one of us, after all the years it took to find each other, got a disease that changed who we were? What if the man of my dreams became someone else?

It soon became apparent that something was seriously wrong with my father-in-law, and we feared it was Alzheimer's. Ray grew more lethargic; he had no interest in things he had previously enjoyed. He became more argumentative, and he started to lose his memories of those he loved. Especially telling was that he could no longer keep track of his grandchildren's names.

We'd heard that Alzheimer's didn't strike people who had active brains and who kept busy as they aged. So we kept thinking, "It couldn't be that." Now we know from personal experience that Alzheimer's can, indeed, strike even those with very active brains and lives.

Finally, the family decided to stop fretting and guessing and to get a diagnosis. Even getting the one we feared would be better than not knowing. So the other siblings decided that, because of location and other circumstances, my husband and I would take Dad to the appointment.

Ray walked into the clinic with a smile on his face. He kept that smile throughout the whole ordeal, and he really worked his charm. He attempted to bluff his way though all the memory questions, but I think he knew he wasn't doing too well. It was trying for him, and as we were leaving he was a little gruff with the receptionist and ornery about getting into the elevator. With a stroke of inspiration I said to him, "Let's go home, Ray. Let's go see Mary Lou." His whole face brightened, and the twinkle returned to his eyes.

"Mary Lou? I love Mary Lou!" he said. Then he calmly stepped into the elevator, and we took him home.

As the disease progressed, my husband's parents had to move from their home of forty-eight years into an apartment in a retirement complex. Later,

Ray moved to an assisted-living facility a few miles away, leaving Mary Lou behind. Although Ray's new home was very nice, it wasn't like living with his wife. Now, he had to wait until she came to see him—and she did, every day. She spent hours visiting with him, checking on him, and helping him to dress, bathe, and eat. She advocated for his best interests, and got him out of the wheelchair and walking down the hall every chance she had.

I noticed that many of the other residents had also had important or exciting careers. There were other attorneys as well as doctors, professors, and all kinds of people who had spent their lives using their minds but now needed others to remind them to eat and to help with the basic activities of daily living. Sometimes I would visit with the other residents while my husband and his mom attended to Ray. I enjoyed chatting with them and helping them in any way I could, but the fear in my heart grew from these encounters. I did not know what I would do if this awful thing happened to my husband and me. What if we lost each other this way?

As time passed, Ray's family continued to love and support him. Still, he drew further and further away from us, and his behavior became increasingly more disturbing. He made odd comments to the other residents, and he resisted directions. I went from being his "girlfriend" to being his "cousin," as, unfortunately, so did all his children and grandchildren.

Despite all that—and despite not being able to hold a coherent conversation with any of us or to do the things that had once defined his life—Ray was in there, somewhere. We just knew it. Sometimes a glimmer of his old sparkle would come back. Sometimes we could see the love in his eyes as he looked at his family while trying futilely to say the appropriate thing. But most of all, we knew he was in there because he never forgot the name of the woman he loved. Even at the very end, he never forgot Mary Lou.

My mother-in-law is eighty-nine years old now. If Ray were alive, they would have been married more than sixty years. She has a heart condition and only part of one functioning kidney. She doesn't complain; she just keeps on living, even though it isn't the same alone. We sometimes talk about Ray, and in those moments, it's as if Mary Lou's beloved husband is still here with her.

As for me, I have less fear now. I have seen through Ray and Mary Lou's example that love remains. Everything else can be taken, but love will remain.

I like to picture Ray, dressed in his finest Navy uniform, waiting on a porch somewhere, just like on their wedding day. Only this time it is he who has gone ahead and is waiting patiently for his bride to join him. I like to think that sometime in the future, Ray will hear the words, "Mary Lou is here. She's come home to you." His face will brighten and his eyes will twinkle, and he'll say, "Mary Lou? I love Mary Lou!" Then Ray and Mary Lou will look into each other's eyes, hold one another, and dance together again, for as long as they wish.

—Deborah Royal

In My Mother's Heart

My mother was diagnosed with Alzheimer's three days after she turned sixty-seven.

My family and I had visited her in her apartment on her birthday. Even though Mom and I lived fairly close to each other, I was busy and preoccupied with my life, and it had been many weeks since I'd been to her home. I noticed it was dark, dusty, and cluttered, which was unusual for the neat-freak that defined my mother's housekeeping personality. She hadn't brushed her hair, either, and she was wearing a tattered nightgown. I wondered why she wasn't dressed, as she'd known we were coming to see her.

"Is everything okay, Mom?" I asked her.

"I'm fine, Janemarie," she said, examining the candle I had bought her. "This is very pretty. Smells good, too."

An hour or so into our visit, her phone rang. It was my Aunt Doris calling Mom to wish her a happy birthday. I tried not to eavesdrop, but that was a difficult feat in such a small apartment.

"No, Janemarie's not here yet," Mom said to Aunt Doris. "I'm expecting her any time, though."

That's weird, I thought. *I'm sitting right here.* I was puzzled but not too concerned.

I decided not to say anything. Shortly after that, we left. "I'll call you tomorrow," I said.

Mom and I called each other every day, despite my occasional irritation. "Mom," I would say, "we never have anything to talk about."

"Sorry I'm being a bother," she would reply. "I just like hearing your voice."

I called her the next evening and the evening after that. On Sunday, it was her turn to call me, which she would do when she came home from church. When the afternoon rolled around without my phone ringing, I called her. It rang and rang. *Maybe she stopped somewhere for lunch*, I thought. I tried calling her a little later. Still no answer. *Maybe she's out shopping.*

When three o'clock came and went without any contact with my mother, I sensed something was terribly wrong, so I drove to her apartment to check in on her. When I arrived, I noticed her car was still in the parking lot. I hurried up the stairs and knocked on her door. "Mom? . . . Mom, are you in there?" I waited for what seemed an eternity before knocking again. When she didn't come to the door, I grabbed her spare key from my purse and let myself in.

I found her on her bathroom floor. "I'm so glad to see you," she said.

I called 9-1-1, and soon police and paramedics joined me by my mother's side.

"You're going to be all right now, Mom," I said. "I love you."

I sped behind the ambulance and joined my mother in the emergency room, where doctors soon realized she had broken her hip.

I used to work in a hospital, so I knew that hip fractures sometimes left patients dazed and disoriented. Often, pain medication was the culprit, so I asked my mother's doctor to discontinue the morphine he had prescribed for her and try something else.

"I think there's something more than that going on," her doctor told me. "Let's focus on her hip for now, and then we'll monitor her condition and run more tests."

My sister and I took turns staying with Mom, because, despite the pain, she kept trying to get out of bed to go to the bathroom. Although she was obviously agitated, she surprised us with the progress she made during physical therapy. We were troubled, however, by her serious state of confusion.

"Do you know where you are?" I would ask her from her hospital room in Cincinnati.

"Why, of course I do," she would say. "I'm in Marion."

I continued, "Do you know what year it is"

"Nineteen-seventy-seven." It was 2002.

At that point, she would usually get cranky and say, "Now stop asking me so many questions! I'm tired, I need a nap."

Every day I awaited a positive change in Mom's mental status. Every day I was sorely disappointed.

Her doctor ordered a series of tests. She failed the mini-mental state examination (MMSE) miserably. Her reflexes, balance, speech, and eye movement seemed a little "off" as well. The doctor finally ordered an MRI, which revealed more about Mom's condition.

"We believe," Dr. Turner said, "that your mother has Alzheimer's. She's probably had it for a while. She was just good at hiding it, and then her hip fracture amplified the symptoms."

I felt like crying. "Will she improve?"

"We'll know more with time," he said.

As the days dissolved into weeks, it became apparent she would be a permanent resident in the long-term care facility near my home. Since there was no longer any need to hold on to her apartment, my sister and I terminated the lease and proceeded to move out her things.

We had last been in her apartment a couple of days after her she was hospitalized, to retrieve some of her clothes and personal care items. At the time, I couldn't help but wonder, *When had she fallen? How long had she awaited rescue from her cold bathroom floor? Several hours? A day or longer?* I dwelled on the unknown more than I should have, and the evidence we had gathered during that quick visit left me wallowing in guilt and regret.

It had been almost six weeks since Mom's fall, and my sister and I had a lot of cleaning and packing to do. Old framed pictures our mother had never bothered to unpack stared back at us, familiar faces that, for whatever reason, Mom had decided not to memorialize on her apartment walls. In her dresser drawers lay childishly scribbled letters from my sister. ("I love you, Mom." "I'm sorry." "You are pretty.") We came upon old stories and personal essays I'd written and shared with my mother. Dozens of Christmas cards and birthday cards and other-occasion cards fell out of dresser drawers. Mom seemed to have saved everything we had ever given her.

Her kitchen revealed a diet consisting of choco-late cupcakes, ice cream, candy, frozen dinners, and coffee. I began piecing together the puzzle of my mother: anxious, sad, bored, and lonely. During the last few years, she had revealed clues that I had obviously ignored. Like a movie, her dark and dusty apartment told a story that evolved as my sister and I cleaned, pitched, and packed. I realized I could have had a lead role in my mother's life story, but, instead, I had opted for a supporting part that didn't even merit a credit at the end. I felt as if I hardly knew anything about her, because I had chosen not to know anything about her.

We spent many more hours sorting through Mom's things and divvying them up into save, donate, and destroy piles. At week's end, we threw a free-for-all moving sale and invited the apartment-complex residents to help themselves. Then we gave the apartment a thorough cleaning and a final inspection.

As we were sorting through Mom's belongings, I found a lock-box that contained important documents, such as her Social Security card, birth certificate, life insurance policy, and a will. The box was crammed with information, so I decided to give it a thorough examination when I returned home. Wedged in the middle of all the documents were two envelopes, one addressed to my sister and the other to me.

I couldn't wait to read whatever was in the envelope, and I almost tore the contents as I ripped it open. It was a letter, dated on my mother's sixty-seventh birthday, that read:

Whenever I celebrate my birthday, Janemarie, my thoughts are with my children. You have given me so much joy, so much love, that you never have any reason to give me a birthday present. The fact that you are my daughter is the best gift in the world.

I don't know where my days will take me, but wherever I go, please understand I carry you in my heart forever. Thank you for just being you.

All my love, Mom.

Tears cascaded down my face.

"What's wrong?" my husband asked me.

"Maybe I'm not such a bad daughter after all," I said. "At least Mom doesn't think so."

I felt relief from my guilt for the first time in weeks, and I was free to love my mother for as long as God decided to share her with me.

The next day, I joined my mom in her room in the nursing home. She had just returned from arts-

and-crafts, and she presented me with a flower pot she had decorated. "This is for you, Janemarie."

Remembering her letter to me, I fought back tears and pointed to a picture I had just hung up on her wall. It was her engagement portrait, circa 1956. The face from the portrait beamed in beauty and love for her soon-to-be husband, my father, who had died in 1968. "Just look at you, Mom. You're gorgeous."

She smiled. "I guess I am."

I positioned the picture so it would be the first thing people saw when they entered her room. I wanted to remind them that this is the woman who awaited their care and attention, that my mother was much more than the confused woman who greeted them from her chair.

I wrapped my arms around Mom in a warm embrace. She hugged me back and said, "Let's go get some dinner. I'm starving!"

—*Jane M. Bratton*

Bedside Stories

Dad sponged down the rails, slats, and sides of the bed, carefully put them together, and tightened the nuts and bolts. He made sure the sides locked and were secure so she wouldn't fall out. He wiped the plastic-covered mattress with soapy water and placed it on the springs, then smoothed the sheets into place. Flower-printed cases enclosed the plastic-covered pillows. Everything was ready. Great Aunt Ann would be comfortably safe.

In the two years since we'd seen Ann at her sister's funeral, she had changed. She was no longer the elegant, six-foot-two Amazon full of energy and drive, her deep hazel eyes sparkling with wit and intelligence. We barely recognized her when she opened the door.

Greasy hair lay in disordered tangles on her shoulders; her mouth was crusted with glazed sugar icing from the crullers she had crammed into her mouth with dirty fingers. The once solid, capable, neatly manicured hands—now knotted with arthritis, the nails chipped and broken—unraveled the loose cashmere threads of a stained cardigan. Her rumpled satin dress smelled of rooms shut away from sun and air for too long. The ripped, ragged hem of a French lace slip straggled over bony knees protruding from wrinkled folds of once full flesh.

Gone was the woman of fashion and intelligence who had turned her personal style into a prosperous chain of beauty salons and who had glided effortlessly and gracefully through the world. Despite her unfashionably ample proportions, with her impeccable taste and sparkling smile, Ann had always looked like she belonged on the cover of a fashion magazine or at the head of an elegant banquet table where she oversaw each tiny detail. Only a bedraggled shadow of her former self remained. Her family dead and gone and her businesses closed, she was living alone in a dark, musty cave of faded elegance.

We took Ann home with us and fit her into our lives. The house was full with my three young boys and me, Mom, Dad, and my sister, Tracy, still living at home, but we were family.

Ann's rich contralto voice with its strength and cultured tones became a querulous nasal whine whenever she wanted something, especially the glazed crullers she preferred over home-cooked food. She wouldn't eat anything else unless Dad gave it to her; she would mumble, grumble, and angrily shake her head whenever anyone else offered her food. Even though he was only her nephew by marriage, his presence calmed her. She trusted him as though he were her father.

Glimmers of the past surfaced like bright, fragile bubbles during the year before Alzheimer's made Ann too weak and fragile to get out of the bed. During that time, her voice gained strength and sureness as she talked of her life, and she seemed to grow younger and younger as she lived her life in reverse. Her eyes, once so wise and intelligent, became more innocent and trusting, empty of cynicism and worldliness as she became a child once again. Photographs and pictures in family albums and books from her library touched some part of her mind hidden in dusty, forgotten corners, and the indulgent smile that had so disarmed and enchanted everyone around her bloomed again. Bony fingers traced perfect, even stitches on embroidered handkerchiefs as though sewing them for the first time. With her movements swift and sure, she would explain the choice of colors and stitches until her eyes dimmed and her hands restlessly plucked at her clothes, lost in a misty fog where the sun didn't reach. A black mink hat with ostrich feathers that curved gracefully down like an exotic veil transported her to the streets of Paris and to a tiny bistro where she dined on fragrant onion soup thick with crusty bread and cheese and sipped a glass of wine. She was there, and then suddenly, she was back.

Ann, always larger than life, became less imposing. Slowly, the wise, knowing light flickered and died, leaving innocence and an artless and open smile. Wisdom gained through decades of work and hard-earned success slowly faltered, fractured, and broke. The layers of her life peeled away until the hard-wired experiences of youth and childhood—lullabies, friendships, nursery rhymes, and quicksilver bursts of laughter—were unearthed and laid bare.

We shared her memories and learned who she was and who she had been. The opening of her first beauty shop, falling in love, and the little moments of her life surprised and delighted us. The confident and self-assured girl she had been now whispered secrets once safely locked away or forgotten. We were with her when she left the small farm where she was born. Her senior dance came alive and faded quickly under a moonlit sky as she got her first kiss.

We relived her first puppy love, her first hat, and her first pair of gloves on an Easter morning when she was five.

Toys appeared from some cobwebbed corner in the attic of her mind alongside crushes on Saturday matinee idols, Christmas trees, Easter bonnets, and white patent leather shoes. Thanksgiving turkeys were fed, killed, cooked, and eaten. We gathered eggs warm from the nest, carried shiny pails of frothy milk, and ate freshly churned butter. Time flashed backward faster and faster until only glimmers of awareness and the sweet, trusting smile of a child remained.

When her body grew feeble, the side rails on her bed stayed up to keep her safe. Her laughter chimed like a silver bell when she saw Dad. When he fed and changed her, she smiled up at him with complete trust. When she no longer recognized Dad's face, she instinctively turned toward the sound of his voice and the touch of his hands like a newborn baby.

Then came the day when Ann became too ill to keep at home, her once strong and sturdy body emaciated and shrunken, her smile and mind gone. She no longer needed the bed in the family room.

Dad dipped the sponge into the soapy bleach water and wiped down the plastic-covered mattress one last time. Carefully taking apart the bed, he washed the railed sides before placing them against the wall. He gathered the parts and carted them into the garage, where he stacked them in the storage area and then went quietly back into the house.

There was more space in the family room with the bed gone, and the room, once filled with the shared memories of a lifetime, echoed with empty silence.

When Ann came to live with us, we got to know her in a way few ever would. She took us on a journey through her life and showed us the sadness and the joy, the trials and the excitement that had led her to the fancy house with expensive furnishings and the closets full of couture clothes, hats, gloves, and accessories. The once formidable Amazon of fashion became, once again, a country girl who delighted in beauty and made it her life.

Had we not tucked her into our lives, we never would have known our great aunt and the world she'd lived in or experienced the wonder of her childhood once again. Most of all, she taught us patience and that, even in the most devastating circumstances, there is still joy.

—J. M. Cornwell

Unchained Memories

"Daggone the doggone luck," Mom crooned with her cool hand on my forehead while I threw up.

As a child, I didn't dream that the doggone luck would ever lead to me taking care of my nurturing mother. Mom was way ahead of me, though, and when I was the right age, she made her wishes plain. A demented old woman we knew had been hauled kicking and screaming from her daughter's to a nursing home. "If I ever get like that, let me kick and scream," Mom said. "Don't let me destroy your family. The mother who took care of you when you were sick and when you had babies and when you broke your elbow never ever wants to live with you."

Her words echoed in my head when her Alzheimer's appeared. All during my childhood it had been a comfort to me that my mother, a nurse who didn't work outside the home, knew what to do about so many things. When I got my smallpox vaccination, Mom knew how to make a "window bandage" to protect the sore without touching it. When our puppy died of rabies after nipping my sister, Mom gave my sister the shots.

She also made things for us. We never questioned how Mom's hand-knit sweaters and caps ended up on Santa's dolls. She taught me to knit, too. At first, she had me make dishrags, because it didn't matter how many mistakes I made on them. Now, I knit Mom's old patterns, and I still wear two of the last sweaters she made.

When I was little, money was tight and my mother didn't think she could sew well enough to risk buying fabric. She would take apart old garments from church rummage sales to make new ones. She had no idea how much harder that was than cutting out fabric from a pattern.

Our family had fun, too. We sang all kinds of songs, from Christmas carols to rounds to silly songs, and all year long we sang old songs, the ones my parents had sung when they were growing up. At home, in the car, and on our family bicycle trip, we sang. Some songs we sang in the same order every time: "Put on Your Old Grey Bonnet," followed by "I Want a Girl (Just Like the Girl)" and "For Me and

My Gal," and ending with "I've Been Working on the Railroad." What we sang wasn't important, but it was always good family time. When we were home, we'd sing around the piano and my dad would play, and we'd usually end up with the same old routine.

One year for Christmas, Daddy went to a Chicago recording studio and recorded himself playing the songs that meant something to us, including the ones we sang together as a family as well as the lullabies he'd played for my sister and me when we were babies. My sister's was Brahms' lullaby. Mine was the angelic theme by Chopin from the B-minor sonata that also contains his famous funeral march. My dad played it by ear, as he played everything else, and the second time through the theme he always flatted a "blue" note, knowing full well it wasn't in the original. As a child I sometimes wept, because it was so beautiful and because I loved my father so much.

The other songs he played on the recording were "Dear Heart" for Mom; "Under His Wings," which his own mother had loved; and a couple of songs he had composed himself, which we all knew and loved. Back then, Daddy had made records for our record players. Later, one of my sons transferred the recordings to tape.

Mom continued to sing joyfully for many years, even though she was developing Alzheimer's. My dad, seeing the early signs of the disease, moved with

Mom from their apartment in St. Louis to an apartment in Bloomington, Indiana, where I lived with my husband. Although I could see her confusion during the process, Mom was still able to adjust to the move, and both my parents lived here happily for three years, until my father died.

For some time after Daddy's death, my mother's understanding of what was happening to her came and went. When it came, it tore her up, because she knew too much, due both to her nursing background and to her sister and grandmother having had Alzheimer's, too.

As her abilities declined, my husband, my son, Joe, and I used her failing eyesight as an excuse to chauffeur her. She mourned the loss of the Buick almost longer than she mourned the loss of her beloved husband.

At first, she was able to live alone, but eventually we had to have someone with her all the time. We were lucky to find a loving friend who did that type of work and to have enough money from my dad's insurance to pay her. Peggy made a tremendous difference, but she couldn't be there nonstop, and no one wanted to work weekends. So Mom became my full-time job, too.

I drove her to the university hospital in Indianapolis, where she was officially diagnosed and started on the last trial of the first drug to be approved by the FDA for the treatment of Alzheimer's. She responded well to the drug, which delayed her decline for some time. The nurse in her was proud to be part of that trial.

For a long time, Mom was able to talk plainly about her wishes. She hoped her body might be useful to medicine after she died. She talked about the end of her life and her wish not to be kept alive after her mind was gone. My sister and I promised to honor her requests.

Some requests were impossible. She begged me to take her "home" . . . "where everyone knows me, and I know everyone." There were many such homes: the tiny town where she'd grown up with her siblings as well as the various towns where my father had been the minister. She had always been at "home" with her church family, whom she worked at knowing and with whom her role was clear. But no such place existed now, because she rarely knew anyone anywhere now. The day her younger sister joined us when we were visiting my sister, near Chicago, Mom took me into the bathroom and asked me who that old woman sitting next to her was.

Sometimes Mom didn't know me. She'd say, "I have to get one of the girls (meaning, me or my sister) to take me to the eye doctor." At first I'd tell her we'd done that and why he couldn't help her eyes. Later, I just agreed.

By then, we'd taken the knobs off the stove, because I'd seen her lighting a cigarette from the gas flame with her hair dangerously close to it. We'd also removed the chair from her outdoor smoking area, to keep hot ashes from burning holes in her clothes.

Mom still had her beautiful white hair styled every week, and she still wore nice clothes, many of which she had made herself after taking a tailoring course. One Sunday, when her eyebrows looked peculiar, it took me a moment to realize that she'd penciled them in with lipstick. I did my best for her with cold cream. Then we left for church with heads held high.

When Mom began to ask the same questions over and over again, my sister and I put together a little book titled "Answers to Your Questions." As her vision declined, we printed it out again in even bigger and bolder type, so she would be able to read it herself. From time to time, we updated the book to add new answers and to simplify the old ones.

The first version began, "You were born in Wadesville, Indiana. You were in nurses training at Welborn Hospital in Evansville." Then it went on to retrace the important steps in her life history and to list her family members and to describe what they were doing now. The book also told her who had died, so that she wouldn't have to keep asking that question and then grieving when she heard the answer. Reading the same thing to herself seemed not to have that effect on her. One section explained why her eyes didn't work right and said that the doctor was sorry he couldn't fix them. Another assured her she had money in the bank and that we paid all her bills with her money.

When she moved to an assisted-living facility that specialized in Alzheimer's care, we added to the book the names of the people who helped her there and something simple about each one.

She read and reread that little booklet many times. Each time, of course, was new. Whenever she questioned the staff, they could say, "Let's see what the book says."

Knowing that the first part of the memoir which she had written before her mind began to fail was the most familiar and meant the most to her, we also printed out that section in big, bold type and gave it to her for Christmas. She was thrilled. She read and reread it. Long after forgetting it was her own story, she would read it and say, "It sounds just like when I was growing up." She enjoyed that story of her own life until she could no longer see well enough to read.

We printed out the whole memoir in regular type for the staff who cared for her. They were impressed to know this woman as an interesting person and as a former nurse rather than only as a patient whose mind was mostly gone.

Mom enjoyed that place till she went to the hospital with a broken hip. The surgery to pin it left her in a great deal of pain. The Alzheimer's disease was so far advanced by then that she couldn't understand where she was or why she hurt so much. Everything bothered her, including the pressure stocking that inflated every few seconds to keep her bad leg from forming a blood clot. Not even her own nursing background helped her. I spent one long day holding her hand and talking softly, but I could not comfort her. Telling her she'd broken her hip and that the doctor had operated to fix it helped only briefly. A moment later, she was lost in misery again.

The next morning, I took her little tape player to the hospital, along with two tapes of my dad playing those old songs on the piano. The first tape was of the record he'd made for us that Christmas long ago. The second tape, made during some holiday get-together, was of the whole family standing around the piano singing.

When I walked into her room, I found Mom sitting up in a chair, crying. I put the first tape into the machine and started it.

She looked up and said, "Is Johnny (her pet name for my dad) here?"

"No," I said. "He couldn't be here, but he wanted you to be able to hear him."

She smiled and started singing the song he was playing, and I joined in. Soon, one member of the nursing staff after another stuck her head in to see who had been put in the room where that pitiful old lady had been. They were surprised to find the same old lady, now anything but pitiful, smiling and singing songs with the man she had loved for nearly sixty years. Her hip must still have hurt, but you couldn't tell it.

Music plus love is a powerful combination.

—*Sara Hoskinson Frommer*

Learning the Rules of the Road

We'd been on the road less than seven minutes when he glanced at his watch. I knew the number of minutes that had passed because I'd been sneaking peeks at the clock on the dash, making bets with myself about how long it would be until he would fidget, squirming and worrying about taking off an entire afternoon, driving away from the demands of his busy car dealerships to take a ride with his daughter.

It was the first time Dad and I had gone anywhere together without my mother or brother and with no business-related side trips—just father and daughter, for an entire afternoon. It was a long time coming. I was forty-one years old, and my father was seventy-one.

"Turn right at this next road," he said, pointing to a narrow county side road up ahead. "I'll show you what used to be a little farming community that soon will be part of progress."

I slowed and made the turn, beginning an afternoon journey that opened a flood of memories my dad shared about his years as a Kansas state-highway commissioner. It would be another seventeen years before I fully understood the importance of that afternoon.

I already knew the ins and outs, the details and hard work, of building car dealerships. They were family businesses, and my brother and I had worked after school, weekends, and summers from the time we were old enough to run errands and wipe down showroom vehicles. But the years Dad simultaneously served as a highway commissioner while building his dealerships were unfamiliar to me. I remembered them primarily as a time of resentment during my youth, because the job had taken even more of my father's time away from us. The real details of highway expansion and road-building were foreign to me.

As I drove along the dirt road, we saw in the distance abandoned farm houses, empty barns, and trees uprooted and lying on their sides. Front loaders and backhoes chewed into land that had been settled by families older than my great-grandparents.

My dad spoke with respect of the hard decisions behind claiming land for public roads, and as we studied the shells of former farms, he recited many of the ancestral lines connected to this land. He told me where some of the owners had moved and how much the state had paid for their land and relocation. It had been many years since he'd been a state-highway commissioner and this had not been one of his projects, yet he'd kept track of some of the families.

As I drove slowly around the highway construction, Dad explained how new highway decisions were made. I learned how commissioners worked with engineers and researchers and legal advisers and how hundred-year flood planes and fair remunerations for condemned property were figured into the equations. From memory, Dad explained the laws and the rules. He cited the specific per-mile cost increases of highway building over several decades, and he knew exactly what could, and could not, be sacrificed for transportation progress.

Homes could be relocated, he said. Farms, too, or portions of acreage purchased for road expansion. Sections of towns could become public domain, if necessary, including private businesses and public buildings, schools, and churches. They were expensive to relocate, though, and had to be carefully and fairly handled.

"But never," he said, and there was a note of pride in his voice, "did I move a cemetery or any portion of a cemetery. Never."

He motioned for me to turn onto a rutted lane, and we crept past highway equipment and around a stand of trees marked for removal. Beyond that, up a slight rise, was a cemetery.

It was very old, with worn headstones we couldn't read until we'd gotten out of the car and walked close to the stones. Several markers were propped up with rocks and surrounded by tall grass and weeds. Others were carefully groomed, with sunflowers or daisies or pansies growing at their bases, and a few had pebbles carefully placed in lines to record the number of visits.

There were less than fifty grave sites in the square plot surrounded by a peeling wooden fence. The three most recent burials had been within the previous decade. The others were dated as far back as the Civil War years, and one stone was so weatherworn that the name and date could not be read. I knelt and ran my fingers over the jagged indentations, trying to make out the names and dates, but the stone kept its secrets. Several markers had epitaphs chiseled in the stone: *Beloved husband and friend. Gone but not forgotten. Served faithfully.*

While I was wandering among the burial plots, Dad had moved to the entrance, where the gate hung on one hinge. He was looking down on the road construction below. When I joined him, he said, "The road's coming along," and pointed off in the distance where the road would attach to another section under construction.

"They did their homework. See?" He pointed specifically to the path cleared in an arc around the rise of ground where we stood. "The irrigation lines for the road won't overflow and flood the cemetery." He gave a low whistle. "That would be a careless mistake, a poor calculation, if the new road changed the drainage and flooded the cemetery. That's how you break trust with families, upending the graves of their loved ones."

While Dad studied the drainage patterns, I watched a bulldozer sever a small farm house. The house was empty, long deserted by its family, but for a moment I glimpsed big blossoms of rose wallpaper on an interior wall. Then it was gone, attacked by a front loader. A pair of dump trucks followed behind for the first loads of debris.

"What about your grandchildren?" I asked, losing patience with my father's preservation of the dead over concern for the living. My daughter was in junior high, and her cousins were in elementary and high school. Dad's grandchildren were the jewels of his life, and he loved them dearly.

"Tell me how it works," I said, "when schools, churches, and homes are uprooted in favor of new roads. Doesn't that break trust with the families?"

One of the hallmarks of my relationship with my father was our verbal sparring. We both loved to argue, to debate issues, possibly because during meals a heated discussion connected us in ways in which we didn't connect otherwise. So I asked the question that day because I wanted to understand the logic behind cool bureaucratic decisions but also to elicit an emotional response from my dad and to prevent him from looking at his watch and deciding it was time to return to the dealership.

He seemed to think for a moment before looking away from the road construction. "You can replace a school, rebuild a church, or design another home to live in. Those are strengths of the living. But a cemetery is different."

Dad squinted at the little cemetery with its rows of headstones and grassy spaces set aside for the next family members. I watched him in profile, seeing his eyes blink and the hard swallow that caught in his throat.

"If you move a cemetery, if you relocate the buried to other locations away from their resting places, how will they be remembered?" he said in hardly more than a whisper.

He paused and gave me a knowing, silent look. One of our frequent and most heated debates had been over my staunch decision to be cremated. Both of us realized, I think, that this was neither the time nor the place to revisit that topic, and without further comment, we went back to the car.

We spent the rest of the afternoon driving along finished highways—including one that Dad had built during his years as commissioner. As I looked at the terrain with fresh eyes, I realized that, where good roads existed, the areas prospered.

We stopped for root beer floats at a small family-owned drive-in, and Dad detailed the steps it had taken to expand the road shoulders so they'd be safer. Up ahead was an elementary school, and beyond that a church and a clinic, with no blind turns in the road and with safe shoulders that had ridges, warning drivers that they'd strayed from the course.

Behind the tree-bordered church was another cemetery. It had been undisturbed by the widening of the road, though I could see that it would have been a logical place to build access to the main highway. Keeping the cemetery separate and building an access farther down the road was a good trade, my dad said.

It was also a good afternoon. Though he had sneaked a few peeks at his watch, Dad didn't suggest we hurry back, and we didn't return home until evening.

For another decade, he went to the main dealership early each morning and put in a long day dealing with second and third generations of car and truck buyers. He took many of the long-time customers home for lunch, and my mother prepared delicious meals, often with vegetables from their garden. Lively, warm conversation was the house specialty.

Then surgery corrected a health problem, but when Dad came out of hours of anesthesia, he was changed. Prior to the operation, we had noticed bouts of confusion, forgetfulness, and irritation, but those escalated from that point on. Every few months, when I drove from Colorado to Kansas to visit, I witnessed increasing symptoms of Alzheimer's that even the best medications and care could not thwart.

My brother finally had to end Dad's involvement in the business. I moved my parents into a nearby full-care apartment, where social interaction was scheduled to keep my mother active, but there were no longer meals grown in the garden or sparkling conversation around a big dining room table. My dad and I no longer debated issues, personal or political.

Now, sometimes in the evening after my mother has gone to bed, I give the caregiver a break and sit beside the hospital bed that prevents bedsores from forming on Dad's shrinking body. If I pat his hand and talk to him, Dad will look away from the television that holds his interest for awhile. He looks at me, and sometimes there's a glimmer of recognition, as though my name or the familiarity of my face or our relationship is almost within his reach . . . almost, but not quite. I tell Dad things, snippets of stories I remember, details of what he ate for dinner, or reminders of visitors who stopped by. Sometimes he listens, squinting like he's trying to connect the dots on a faded page. Other times, he waves me out of the way so he can see the television screen. Cooking shows are among his favorites, though as far as I know he's never cooked a meal on his own in his entire adult life.

What I have repeatedly told him, as I sit beside him and pat his arm, is about the day we spent an entire afternoon together and went for a drive. I tell him how grateful I am that he educated me on the rules of road building. I also tell him that the same cemetery rule he never broke as a commissioner has now become my promise to him. His final resting place will not be moved, not for a road or for progress or for any reason. I assure my father that even though he might not know where or who he is, others will not forget.

—Marylin Warner

The Card

Holding and turning it over in my hand, I open the envelope and pull out the card to read the words, "You're not just a special daughter; you're a very unique woman we are proud of." I view the signature: "Love, Helen and James." Tears tumble.

My mind launched back to the afternoon when, in an eye-opening moment, my mother realized she hadn't purchased birthday cards for my sons. All her life, Mother had been all about sending cards and notes—to encourage friends, to celebrate each family member's milestones, to offer words of comfort from home to new college students. Her connection to others was her keen ability to sense when someone needed a card of cheer.

So, in their early years, my boys had grown up anticipating the regular-as-clockwork cards from

Grandma and Grandpa. Valentines, Easter greetings, Halloween notes, and birthday cards, always with a check tucked inside, were found in the mailbox. As teenagers, they'd even laughed when some of those cards were bedecked in flowery pastels, teapots, or butterflies rather than more traditional masculine images. They understood Grandma was struggling with the frustrating changes of living with Alzheimer's disease. Even as the signatures grew sloppier, they took it all in stride. As busy teens, they might not have even missed getting a card at all this year.

But from a grandmother's perspective, this situation was dire. She had sent cards her entire life—and she was *not* going to ignore the boys' birthdays next year! Determination gleamed in her eyes as she voiced her intent to purchase cards. I offered to drive both my parents to a nearby drug store to accomplish her mission, and we headed out in that direction.

Although still ambulatory, my parents' pace has slowed to what seems like a snail's pace to me. Not long ago I remarked to a friend that going somewhere with them was like shifting a manual transmission car from fifth gear to first without downshifting through the gears in between. I find it very challenging to move slowly, for my life consists of various modes of multitasking. However, I deliberately slowed my pace that day as I watched Dad help

Mother from the car and as, together, they moseyed toward the store entrance.

Once inside, I watched as they edged toward the card aisle. Card shopping was foreign territory to my father, who normally ventured only into grocery stores. Personal greeting card selection had been Mother's realm, not his. Recognizing her continued dependency and her sense of urgency, his shaking hand gently moved to the center of her back as he guided her. Gently, he brought the love of his life to the right section, edging her away from the pink, floral cards.

Although I felt awkward at first, I eventually jumped in to assist them in finding two cards that would work for my sons. Since Mother no longer carried a purse, I made sure my dad had enough cash. There had been several times in recent months when he'd run short. For years, he had depended upon my mother to bring along sufficient money for their needs. However, as life was changing, they were adapting as best they could.

Back in the front seat of the car, Mother carefully began signing the cards. Many questions were asked about which card was for which boy and how to sign. "Should I put Helen and James?" she asked innocently.

I blinked. "Grandma and Grandpa would work fine," I quietly responded.

She carefully turned the pen over, not sure how to twist it open. Gently, I reached over and guided her hand. I turned my head to look out my window. Realizing this entire set of simple tasks was beyond her current abilities, I found myself biting my lip in both frustration and disbelief. Sure, I'd realized she wasn't able to enjoy many of her former activities, but somehow I'd missed the fact that she could no longer even sign her name without assistance. Shrugging off my gloomy thoughts, with a quick smile I explained that I would be glad to keep the cards in a safe place until the time arrived for the boys' birthdays—knowing that she was well beyond the capability of addressing them and mailing them in a timely manner. As we sat together in my car, I found myself essentially questioning life's value for her.

Suddenly, as though a light bulb had gone off inside her brain, Mother jerked her head toward me. "When is your birthday?" she asked.

I responded that mine was situated between that of my two boys. Looking down at the duo of cards in her lap, she replied simply, "We must get a card for you."

Back into the store we ambled, this time with Dad gently steering Mother toward the pink section. If I'd thought it was awkward watching card selection for my children, it was certainly more so when I was the intended receiver. I felt unable now to hold back the tears. Never would I have anticipated the indescribable, gut-wrenching knots associated with observing something so simple taking such incredible concentration and effort. However, with sheer determination, she personally selected one and headed off with Dad to the counter. I lunged toward the door.

Once outside, I gulped in a ragged breath of fresh air. Somehow, I had to get through the next few minutes as well. I didn't want Mother to realize that her slowness of mind was painful for me to watch. How could I explain that this challenge hurt me greatly? Would my parents even understand if they saw tears in my eyes?

Fortunately, I found some tissues in the glove box and treasured a few precious moments alone to gather my composure. I watched them saunter back to the car for a second time, Dad again holding the door to the front seat for Mother. Once she was comfortably seated, I handed her my pen. She meticulously opened the card, signed it, and sealed the envelope.

"I'll keep this one with the others," I said, as she silently handed it my way.

So it came to be that on July 27, I opened the birthday card that was filled with meaning. I'd opened all the other cards from family and friends as they had arrived, but I'd held this one, from my mother, until the actual date of my birth. Toward the end of a day filled with various special surprises and moments of celebration, I quietly slipped back to the room where I'd tucked the card.

This birthday, I have been abundantly blessed by the tender love shown by a simple green and pink card, signed in barely legible script, "Helen and James." No, they are not "Helen and James" to me. They are Mother and Dad, as they always will be. No matter how sloppy the signature, no matter what comes down the pike in the months ahead, no matter if this is the last card my mother ever gives me, I know that I am and forever will be well loved.

—*Yvonne Riege*

The Answer Is Tom Cruise

"I think Tom Cruise is the answer," my dad says.

We are sitting in my mom's room in the Alzheimer's unit. Dad and I are perched on the bed; Mom sits in a chair, bent over a photo album.

Was it only last month that she looked at the pictures as though she might actually recognize the people in them? Now, even with all of our pointing and exaggerated enthusiasm, she barely notices the people underneath the plastic covering. She does notice the plastic covering and picks at a corner of it.

"Tom Cruise?" I ask. "Tom Cruise is the answer to what?"

Dad nods sagely and tells me this story:

One night my parents were celebrating their forty-somethingeth wedding anniversary in one of Memphis's older and finer restaurants. They were seated at a quiet corner table, when a fluttering of people, a craning of heads, and a rising level of conversation prompted them to look around and spot a handsome man striding through the restaurant. He seemed to have an entourage surrounding him, but he stopped to shake hands and sign napkins. Then he smiled, waved to the restaurant at large, and let himself be ushered into a private room.

"That Tom Cruise is one handsome man," Mom said as she and Dad settled back to their meals.

Dad looked up. He and Mom often discussed movies, but he had never heard her speak so definitively about a man's good looks.

"Shall I try to get him to come over and talk with us?" he asked. He was already planning just how he would make the approach—a private conversation with the waiter, who was already charmed by the length of their marriage. That conversation would lead to a more conspiratorial tête-á-tête with the aloof maître 'd, with occasional references to my mother, silver haired and looking beautifully angelic as she nibbled on her salmon bérnaise.

"Oh, no," Mom said. "I don't want to talk to him. I just want to look at him."

Now, fifteen years after the almost-encounter with Tom Cruise, my dad is considering Mr. Cruise as one in a series of possible saviors—people, places, or events that can release my mother from her Alzheimer's prison and liberate her back into the woman she used to be.

"I believe when your mother sees Tom Cruise on the screen, she will know who he is and remember that evening we saw him," Dad tells me, as we watch Mom get up to fold and refold a pillowcase.

She pulls the blue, ribbed bedspread half up on the other bed, then sits down, then stands up, then pulls on the bedspread again. "Do you want this?" she asks me, with a tone of exasperation in her voice.

"No," I say. "I don't need it. You can leave it right there."

Mom puts her hands on her hips, then leans down to pick up a piece of lint from the floor.

"Mom doesn't even know who *I* am half the time," I tell my father. "I am going to be very upset if she recognizes Tom Cruise. Plus, he could look different on the movie screen."

"I think she will recognize him," Dad says.

Dad tells me his plan: He envisions making a preliminary phone call to the manager at a nearby theater. "I am an older man. I am bringing my wife to the movies. But she's easily distracted and may not stay long. If she has to leave early, I'd like to arrange in advance for a refund," my dad plans on saying. If the movie is a failure, at least it will not cost too much.

The last time my mom went to the movies, she bolted out of the theater just after the opening credits and strode off into another theater. I followed her inside, where she spent ten minutes fiddling with the stuffing that was oozing out of the seats. Then she left that theater. She and I walked up and down the corridors and ate popcorn while Dad finished watching his movie.

"I don't think Mom can sit still even while she's waiting for the movie to start," I say to Dad. "I don't think she'll notice the screen. She doesn't even focus on the television when it's on."

"Perhaps we just haven't found the right movie. I believe that when she sees Tom Cruise, she'll remember how she used to like him. She'll remember almost meeting him. She'll sit and watch the movie."

Meanwhile, Mom sits on the bedspread and reaches under her orange stretch pants to explore the top of her adult diaper. Then she tugs again at the spread. "What the heck is this?" she says. "It's candled, you bums."

I watch my dad. He explains to Mom it's a bedspread. He reminds her of the bedspread they had years ago, a beautiful ivory coverlet that my grandmother had crocheted.

My mom sits still while he talks, then resumes her yanking. "So and so's," she says.

"I'm going to get a newspaper, see what the movie times are," Dad tells me. "Will you stay here with your mother?"

I watch my Dad walk out of the room.

The head nurse will find him a paper. Maybe she will raise her eyebrows when she hears his plan. Maybe she will just nod and smile. She is used to my father's ideas and schemes.

"Your father is often unrealistic," she once told me.

"I know," I said. "I like that about him."

"I do, too," she said.

Like me, she secretly wants one of these schemes to work. My father has a blindness that is of the heart, not of the eyes. He refuses to give up on the woman he has loved for so many years. Of course, he knows Mom has Alzheimer's. But he believes that she can overcome it. She has overcome so much in her life; why not this?

He comes back with the paper.

"The movie is at that little theater, just ten minutes away. I think this could work. Right, Frannie?" he asks, raising his voice to get Mom's attention.

She looks up from opening the drawer and turns to my father as if he is a sudden full moon.

"Right," she says.

"Maybe you should walk in late, after the movie has started, so Tom might be already on the screen," I say, a spot of hope rattling around in me.

"Yes, that's a good idea," Dad says. "I'll bring a flashlight and guide us to our seats."

"Do you want me to come with you?" I ask.

"No, I think your mother and I need to do this together. We'll be fine. Won't we, Frannie?"

"Whatever," Mom says, grabbing a fistful of her shirt.

Later that night, I get a call from Dad.

"Well?" I ask, hoping that something miraculous happened.

"Tom was on the screen when we walked in, and I think she smiled. But I'm not sure she recognized him, with the make-up and different hair and such. And she didn't seem to understand how to sit down in the seats, so we left."

"Did you get your money back?"

"We got all our money back," Dad tells me proudly. "You know, I think you were right. She needs to see Tom Cruise in person. I'm going to call a promoter I know in Memphis and see if he can give me a lead . . ."

I smile as I listen to Dad's newest plan. He has an energy and a sense of hope in his voice that I haven't heard in months. I guess Tom Cruise is an answer, if not for my mother then at least for my dad.

—Deborah Shouse

This story was first published in the author's book, Love in the Land of Dementia: Finding Hope in the Caregiver's Journey, *Creativity Connection Press, August 2006.*

Radiance in the Waning Light

"I have had a good life," my father says. A full sentence, all words in place.

"You've had a long life," I say.

He looks at me in surprise. "I have? How long?"

"Eighty-five years."

"Eight-five," he says and rubs the stubble on his chin. "Really?"

We sit together on the deck of a small cottage my parents have rented for the past forty-nine Fourth of Julys. In the late afternoon sunlight, I survey the Minnesota lake before us, the water as green as the Squirt bottles my dad pulled out of pop machines for me long ago. Boats rush by, leaving the roar of their motors to meld with the sounds of glee generated from children pushing one another from the swimming raft. My mother and youngest son fish from the dock.

"You don't have to sit with me," he says.

"I know."

"How old again?"

"Eight-five."

He shakes his head and smiles.

He's right. I don't have to sit here, but it is for moments like this that I do. During the six years my father has been slipping away due to the effects of Alzheimer's, I have sought these snippets, discovering them in the hiding place that has taken him. Even though it is easier to focus only on tending to his care, I yearn for these rare moments when he is still my dad and I am still the daughter. Experiencing those connections are well worth the wait, even when it means sitting next to him while the leaves rustle in the trees above and while a world he is now only a small part of glides by like the lone canoe out on the water.

Fourteen-hundred miles separate me from my parents. I spend extended stays with them throughout the year—several weeks at Christmas, a month in the summer—but it is difficult, as I am still raising a family.

My eighty-one-year-old mother is my father's lone caregiver. Although a breast cancer survivor—twice—she has been blessed with manageable illnesses. But my father's needs are increasing. His eyesight is almost gone. His size 14 EE feet are cradled in the thickest soled and sturdiest of shoes; his large hands have difficulty with buttons and zippers, and his food needs not only to be prepared, but also finely cut, even finer than my children's when they were babies. He rises from a chair using both hands and stands a while to steady himself before stepping forth, cane in hand. With wary eyes I follow his labored steps, wondering whether he will arrive at his destination and how much longer he will be able to walk.

At each visit I see the debilitation, the subtle and not-so-subtle changes: The further deterioration of his speech and memories. The staring at the family photos on the wall as he strains to place the names of his children and grandchildren with their pictures. His need to follow the news of the day, to keep himself in this world. His being aware and yet unaware that he can no longer make the big decisions and that his self-sufficiency was ebbing away.

We have arrived at a time when changes are inevitable: Safer housing than a two-story home. More caregiving. Adjustments in clothing—Velcro fasteners and elastic waistbands. Simpler meals— more grilled cheese sandwiches and meat loafs. One can only imagine my father's thoughts at having to leave his home, at the possibility of being separated from his wife, and at the loss of so many things that give definition and purpose to a man's life—fruitful employment, the now unusable driver's license, the ability to make his own sandwich and to concentrate well enough to read a book or watch a movie or to remember where it is he is going that day.

This fall I returned to my parents' house for a week because my mother was ill. I was the third of four children to take a week's turn at staying with and looking after my parents. Aside from making sure they had three good meals and snacks in between, clean sheets and laundry, I found myself reminding my dad to brush his teeth, explaining each day that it needed to be done morning and night. I helped when his pants didn't go smoothly over his feet. He asked me to clip his fingernails. I took him for a haircut and then to have the wax removed from his ears (so he could still say "What?" to my mother and grin when she looked away). I walked with him to the end of the street twice a day. Each time as we came out of the front door, I retold the strategy—what to hang onto, where to step down, when to step forward. Each time.

Every day, many, many times a day, he expressed his concern for who would take care of them when I left. Finally, two days before my departure, I thought to write it out for him. He fingered the pages I had written in large letters, listing the days of the week followed by the name of the caregiver. The day before I was to leave, my brother, Jim, would arrive for eight days, followed by a visiting nurse for two days; then my mother would be well. By writing it out for him, he no longer asked me over and over, but I knew he was still unsure. He worried what would happen if Mom didn't get well. I didn't know how to write that answer on a sheet of paper in large print.

I had an early morning flight, so the night before when my dad got ready for bed, he collected me in his large grasp. He had tears in his eyes, and, of course, I could not contain mine. We couldn't look at each other, which is not unusual for the two of us.

"Be good. Do well. I love you," he said.

I couldn't say anything.

We survived that, and he went to the kitchen table to eat a bowl of corn flakes with a banana that my brother had set out for him. I retreated into the depths of my mother's lounger.

When Dad finished his snack, he stood and walked toward me, motioning with his hand. "Come."

I went to him, and we met halfway. I'm not sure who held up whom, but the hug he gave me was my dad's hug. He still knew what I needed.

"It will be okay," I said.

"I've lived a good life," he says.

"A long one," I say.

"How long again?"

"Eighty-five years. You want me to write it down?"

"Please."

He looks at the paper in his hand and smiles. "Eighty-five," he says, tracing the big eight and five printed on the sheet. "Eighty-five."

A good, long life, indeed.

—Julie Sucha Anderson

Around the Corner

A diagnosis is waiting for us, hovering around the corner. My mother's internist mentioned it, once, about four years ago. "I think you have a touch of Alzheimer's," she told my mother, who then promptly forgot that she'd ever heard those words.

But I haven't forgotten. I've been holding that word in my pocket these past four years, keeping it close and occasionally pulling it out, like a crumbled receipt or old movie ticket, as an explanation for all that goes wrong. But I haven't wanted to really examine it. I haven't gone for a second opinion or made an appointment for a neurologist or investigated the local clinic that specializes in, er, that disease.

What good would it do to put my mother through tests that she would fail? To give her an official stamp? What if it turned out to be definitively

positive? Then what would I do? And if it were nega-
tive? Would we do anything differently than we're
doing now?

Medications? They are, in spite of the marketing
enthusiasm of pharmaceutical ads, woefully ineffec-
tive, except for people who are "on the brink."

"We need to wait," says my physician husband.
"For the point when she can't do her ADLs." I
remember that acronym from my old physical therapist days. ADL: activities of daily living.

My mother is still independent when it comes to
bathing. She draws a steaming hot bath every night
and climbs in unassisted. She dresses herself, albeit
in slightly stained shirts that she favors for eight days
in a row. She combs her hair, although she sometimes looks like Einstein's sister. She's managing her
ADLs just fine.

But not everything is manageable. Recently
she called out because she could not figure out how
to make a phone call. Often she cannot open an
umbrella. There is no way she can operate our high-
tech television, with its receiver, separate screen, and
cable box. She can't drive a car anymore. She absolutely cannot set the temperature or timer on our
oven. She can, however, still work the microwave.

She can sort the recycling and remember to bring
it up to the garage on Wednesday nights. She can

cook rice, which she does pretty much every night. I call in from on the road, on the way home, and she asks, "Shall I start the rice?" She can walk the wobbly dog several times a day. She can converse with the next-door neighbors, who adore her. When I take her to my office, she can affix labels and stamps to envelopes. But she can't use a calculator—she, who kept my father's financial records meticulously organized, who worked for years as a bookkeeper for the National Council of Churches in Manhattan.

It is hard to stay patient and compassionate and to fight back feelings of stunned incredulity when she says, "I don't know how to do this." The other members of my family—my two daughters and husband—are better equipped than I am to face her condition. I confess that sometimes I snap at her. Sometimes I lose it and say, "Don't you remember?" No. She doesn't.

This is my mother—the woman who, pretty much, raised me alone while my father traveled through ten states on his sales business. (He was home a grand total of twelve weeks a year, which to him was a generous "vacation time," but in retrospect, left her as a virtual single mother.) She shoveled the snow from the driveway and raked mountains of leaves from the half-acre yard. She worked in the front office at my elementary school, and at night she sat at the dining room table with towering piles of "paperwork." I remember the sound of the adding machine, trilling like a third heartbeat through the house. When the hot water heater exploded, she dealt with it.

It is hard to take when my mother asks the same question twelve or fifteen times and to answer it gently, as if it is the first time. "When is Mollie coming home?" "Tuesday night." Twenty minutes later. "When is Mollie coming home?"

My daughters will answer those questions a hundred times if they must, and they do not roll their eyes or heave sighs from their chests. It doesn't make them angry or sad or frustrated. This is just Nana. They love her. She asks questions; they answer.

It's different for me. I want to know where my mother went, the tough little woman who could do anything. She trained to be an emergency medical technician when she was sixty years old. She leaped into a pool and learned how to deliver a baby on a sidewalk. She could swim miles in choppy ocean water. She always beat me at racquetball.

She is still tough. For an eighty-four-year-old woman, she can still accomplish amazing things. She bowls. She quilts. She makes rice. She walks two miles downhill to town to buy herself a candy bar at the drugstore, and she walks two miles back up. She cracks jokes and goes to basketball games, following the orange ball with rapt attention.

I think I live with a lot of fear, and fear makes me angry. I fear losing her, to death or dementia. I fear that one day she won't wake up. I fear that one day she won't remember my name.

I went away for a weekend not long ago, and when I came back, she said, "I missed you." She gave me a ragged little hug, something that was not a frequent occurrence during my childhood. I took it, and it felt good.

The uncertainty is hard to live with. But it's really all we have. I don't know if she's just getting older or if that scarlet A has embroidered itself into her brain. Part of me doesn't want to know. Time marches on, and around the corner it will tell us, or maybe it won't. We'll continue to live each day, taking care of each other, making memories that one day we'll all, eventually, relinquish. But for now, I hold them tight, here in my pocket.

—Susan Ito

This story was first published in the electronic magazine, Literary Mama.

Contributors

Julie Sucha Anderson ("Radiance in the Waning Light") lives in Austin, Texas, with her husband and three sons. A novel and essay writer, she is the co-editor of *Grrl Talk: Sass, Wit, and Wisdom from the Austin WriterGrrls.* Her work has appeared in many publications, including *Mom Writers Literary Magazine,* ThisIBelieve.org, and Austin-Mama.com.

Mitzi L. Boles ("A Timeless Gift") lives in Payson, Arizona, with her husband and daughter. She has a bachelor's of arts degree in journalism and has spent nearly twenty years working in the field of education and for local news media outlets. She shares her passion for writing with wildlife rescue and is currently working on a series of children's books about wildlife conservation.

Laura L. Bradford ("Only Love Remains") is a writer, residing in Walla Walla, Washington. She seeks to encourage others by sharing her experiences during thirty years as a caregiver. You can find more of Laura's stories in *Chicken Soup for the Father and Son Soul* and the Life Savers for Women book series.

Jane M. Bratton ("In My Mother's Heart"), a graduate of Ohio State University, has been published in the *Cincinnati Enquirer* and *34ᵗʰ Parallel* magazine. She currently works for a public university in Kentucky, where she resides with her husband and two children.

Jenoa Briar-Bonpane ("To Be Present") is a writer, therapist, consultant, and mother who lives on the lost coast of Northern California with her husband and two mighty daughters.

Virginia McGee Butler ("Forgetting, Remembering"), a retired teacher, does freelance writing in Hattiesburg, Mississippi. Her writing has been published in *Once Upon a Time*, *Highlights for Children*, *A Cup of Comfort® for Sisters*, *The Delta Kappa Gamma Bulletin*, and other publications. For fun, she gardens, plays word games, and still sews invisible hems.

Ann Campanella ("The Other Woman") is a mother who writes poetry and creative nonfiction in her spare time. Her poetry collection, *What Flies Away* (Main Street Rag Publishing Company), shares the grief and redemption of her mother's descent into Alzheimer's. Campanella lives in Huntersville, North Carolina, with her husband and daughter.

J. M. Cornwell ("Bedside Stories") is a nationally syndicated journalist, writer, book reviewer, and editor who lives in the Colorado Rockies. Her work has appeared in the Chicken Soup and Cup of Comfort book series, *Ohio Magazine*, and many other national and regional publications. Her personal blog is called Cabin Dreams.

Barbara Davey ("Teaspooned Victories") is the vice president of marketing and public relations at Christ Hospital, Jersey City, New Jersey. Whenever time permits, she can be found in the hospital's sub-acute care unit, where the majority of patients are afflicted with Alzheimer's disease. She and her husband, Reinhold Becker, live in Verona, New Jersey.

Suzanne Endres ("Going Home") loves to write. She has a horse, a pug, and three cats. Suzanne earned her bachelor's and master's degrees at Eastern Washington University. She lives in Washington, but her heart longs for her real home in her birth state, Idaho. Her family often stays there in their cabin.

Barbara Jeanne Fisher ("It Isn't the End of the World") and her husband live in Fremont, Ohio, where she owns the Open Book store. She is the author of the novel *Stolen Moments,* is published in eight of the Chicken Soup for the Soul series, and is the editor of *Voices of Alcohol* and *Voices of Lung Cancer.* She has also published two children's books, *How Much Can Teddy Bear?* and *Nobody's Lion.*

L. S. Fisher ("You're Going the Wrong Way") is an office manager in Sedalia, Missouri. A longtime Alzheimer's Association volunteer and advocate, she was the project leader and editor of *Alzheimer's Anthology of Unconditional Love.* Widowed with two sons and four grandchildren, she writes short stories for relaxation.

Sara Hoskinson Frommer ("Unchained Memories") is the author of *Death Climbs a Tree, Witness in Bishop Hill, The Vanishing Violinist, Murder & Sullivan, Buried in Quilts,* and *Murder in C Major.* She lives with her husband, Gabe, a retired professor of psychology at Indiana University, in Bloomington, Indiana. They have two sons, Charles and Joe.

Nancy C. Gerth ("Sign Here, Please") lives on the top of a mountain in Idaho, where she splits wood, helps repair bulldozers, and writes back-of-the-book indexes for publishers all over the world.

Tanya Ward Goodman ("The Bird House") is a freelance writer and full-time mother. She lives in Los Angeles, California, with her family. She is currently working on a memoir chronicling her experience with her father and grandmother during their simultaneous battles with Alzheimer's disease.

Valerie Kay Gwin ("Good Medicine") works as an administrative assistant at an educational service unit. She and her husband live in Kearney, Nebraska, and have one son, who is in college. She is a freelance writer and an active member of a local Christian writers group. Another of her stories appears in A Cup of Comfort® for Grandparents.

Erika Hoffman ("Lest We Forget, Thank You") is a retired teacher, mother of four, Duke University graduate, wife, and resident of Chapel Hill, North Carolina. As she cares for her elderly father, she is penning her first novel—a thriller set in Piedmont.

Loraine J. Hudson ("My Mother's House") lives in Eagle, Michigan, with her husband, daughter, and assorted animals. She works full-time at Michigan State University. When she isn't writing, she enjoys doing stained glass, gardening, and riding her retired racehorse. She is the author of a series of middle grades light fantasy books written under the pseudonym Judith Wade.

Susan Ito ("Around the Corner") lives in California. She coedited A Ghost at Heart's Edge: Stories & Poems of Adoption (North Atlantic Books). Her writing has appeared in

Growing Up Asian American, Hip Mama, Making More Waves, the Bellevue Literary Review, and *CHOICE.* She is a columnist and creative nonfiction co-editor at *Literary Mama,* an e-zine.

Christine Kiley ("The Connection") lives in Milan, Ohio, with her husband, Brian, and their three teenage children. She graduated from Ohio State University and has been a school nurse for sixteen years.

Jennifer Kuskovski ("Lost and Found") is an elementary school teacher in Minneapolis. She sends her best to all Alzheimer's families, who are on their own personal journeys of reconnecting and getting to know loved ones in a new way.

Sue Fagalde Lick ("Respite from the Storm"), a former newspaper editor, has published countless articles, short stories, and poems, plus three books on Portuguese Americans and a writer's guide called *Freelancing for Newspapers.* She and her husband, Fred, who is in the middle stages of Alzheimer's disease, live in South Beach, Oregon.

Alison Jane Light ("Sweets for the Journey") is a freelance copywriter and a self-confessed travel addict. She has written a book on Peruvian cuisine and currently lives in Brussels with her husband and son, where she writes, cooks, and has developed a firm belief in the restorative powers of chocolate.

Sherry Matthews ("Doing Our Best"), a native of Texas, now lives in El Sobrante, California. An administrative assistant, she has also worked as a commercial artist and a medical assistant. The mother of one daughter, Sherry enjoys drawing, reading, and listening to music, but writing, above all, is her favorite pastime.

May Mavrogenis ("Where Are We Going?") is a retired French teacher living in New York. Her cats have been treated for nervous breakdowns but are recovering. Her story "Vindication" is published in A Cup of Comfort® for Grandparents.

Laurie McConnachie ("Lost in the Moment") is a writer who enjoys exploring the nature of life through her work and has numerous publishing credits. She holds a bachelor's of arts degree and a master's of arts degree in art history and art education from Stanford University. She lives in Seattle with her husband and wee son. Laurie dedicates this essay to her dynamic and loving father—truly an unforgettable man.

Camille Moffat ("The Triumph of Love") lives in the Blue Ridge Mountains overlooking the Shenandoah Valley. A writer and astute people watcher all of her life, she says, "My problem is that I think too much." To date, that problem has not been rectified.

Kathleen M. Moore ("I Am My Mother's Daughter, After All") lives in Minneapolis, Minnesota, and works as a budget analyst for the county. Her nonfiction publications include stories about her time in Ethiopia as a Peace Corps volunteer, being a single mother, and teaching English to immigrant women newly arrived in Minneapolis.

Debbie Mumford ("Close Call") lives in Vancouver, Washington, with her husband of more than thirty years, a ghost-white cat, and a toasted-marshmallow colored mastiff. Her short fiction has appeared online in Flash Me Magazine, KidVisions, and Dragons, Knights & Angels. She has several novels available online from Freya's Bower.

Connie L. Peters ("I Can Chase Lions") and her husband live in Cortez, Colorado, where they care for a woman with developmental disabilities. They have two grown children. Connie's nonfiction, poetry, and children's fiction has appeared in many publications. She teaches Story Express, a monthly creative writing class to homeschoolers.

Gail Pruszkowski ("In the Valley of Denial") is a lifelong resident of Philadelphia, Pennsylvania. She works as a drafting supervisor while pursuing her love of reading, writing, and reviewing for *Romantic Times BOOKreviews* magazine. She shares her life with three children, five grandchildren, two Tonkinese cats, and one patient husband, who rarely sees her without a book in hand.

Lydie Raschka ("Sand"), a Michigan native, lives in Manhattan with her husband and son. She works as a freelance writer and on-again, off-again Montessori teacher-trainer. She has written essays for *Salon*, the *Christian Century*, and the *New York Times*.

Yvonne Riege ("With a Spring in Her Step" and "The Card") is an ordained Church of the Brethren pastor, residing near Wakarusa, Indiana. She and her husband, Mark, have fun traveling and interacting with their two teenage sons. She enjoys playing jazz vibes and auxiliary percussion in various local settings. When relaxing, she can usually be found nestled up with a good read.

S. Ann Robinson ("Loss, Love, and Acceptance") worked for four decades as an instructor, business manager, seminar leader, staff writer, wife, and mother. She now lives in Northern Virginia, where she teaches at the local community college, attends American Sign Language classes, writes for regional publications, and enjoys nurturing her granddaughter, Victoria.

Deborah Royal ("Waiting for Mary Lou") is a former early childhood educator. She lives with her husband, Bill, in beautiful Bellingham, Washington. Between them, they have eight grown children. Deborah enjoys dancing, walking, working with crafts, making up stories with some of her eight grandchildren, teaching classes on various subjects, and attending book club and writers' group. This is her third published story.

Deborah Shouse ("Wanted: Another Mother" and "The Answer Is Tom Cruise") is a speaker, writer, and editor from Prairie Village, Kansas. Her writing has appeared in *Reader's Digest, Newsweek,* and *Spirituality & Health.* She is donating all proceeds from her book *Love in the Land of Dementia: Finding Hope in the Caregiver's Journey* to Alzheimer's programs and research.

Anne-Christine Strugnell ("The Same, Only Different") is a professional writer (who sometimes writes as Meridian James) and amateur mother living in Marin County, California. Her work has been published in *A Cup of Comfort® for Writers* and in magazines serving the high-tech industry and has aired on National Public Radio. She dedicates this story to her siblings and to Tom, her mother's partner.

Samantha Ducloux Waltz ("Tell Me Not to Worry") is a freelance writer in Portland, Oregon. Her essays can be seen in the Cup of Comfort and the Chicken Soup book series as well as in other anthologies. She has also published adult nonfiction and juvenile fiction under the names Samantha Ducloux and Samellyn Wood.

Marylin Warner ("Learning the Rules of the Road") lives with her husband, Jim, near the Garden of the Gods in Colorado Springs, Colorado, where her father, Ray Shepherd, loved to visit. Marylin is a freelance writer and a teacher and workshop leader for adult writing groups. As the "Mor-Mor" of wonderful grandchildren, she's recently published several children's stories.

Jeanne Wilhelm ("Strawberries in January") is a retired hospice nurse turned writer, living in central Pennsylvania. A member of the West Branch Christian Writers, she is a regular contributor to *The Season's Meaning*. Her faith and family give purpose to her life. Gardening and endurance hiking add beauty and excitement. She recently completed Hike for Discovery in the Colorado Rockies.

Renea Winchester ("One Brief Moment") is a freelance writer who splits her time between the mountains of North Carolina and Atlanta, Georgia. She writes fiction and nonfiction. Her work earned the Appalachian Writers Association Award and has appeared in *Birds and Blooms*.

Kathleen McKenzie-Winn ("Apple, Hat, Ashtray") lives in Prairie Village, Kansas. She worked as a paralegal in the mortgage lending business for many years but is now a full-time freelance writer. Kathleen has been published in the *Kansas City Star* and *Newsweek Magazine*. She is currently working on a book related to her family's experience with Alzheimer's disease.

About the Editor

Colleen Sell has compiled and edited more than twenty volumes of the *Cup of Comfort*® book series. A veteran writer and editor, she has authored, ghost-written, or edited more than a hundred books; published scores of magazine articles and essays; and served as editor-in-chief of two award-winning magazines, associate editor of a national business magazine, and home and garden columnist of a regional newsmagazine. She and the love of her midlife, T. N. Trudeau, share a turn-of-the-century farmhouse on forty acres in the Pacific Northwest.